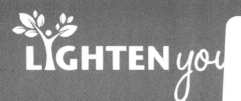

Animal,
Vegetable,
CRIMINAL.

HOW CORPORATE GREED
IS BUYING OUR GOVERNMENT
AND STEALING YOUR HEALTH

Colleen Patrice, M.A.

For Brett.
You are my Foundation, my Support, and my Ballast.
Words cannot convey how Immensely Grateful I am for You,
and how Incredibly Rich My Life Is with You in it.

ACKNOWLEDGMENTS

It *truly* takes a village. Without the incredible support of my family, friends, and pre-publication team, this book would not be in your hands.

My heartfelt appreciation to:

Momma Sue and Gene Bean, who, since the day I met them, have always provided a loving, stable, secure place for me to land… in heart and home. I can't imagine where I'd be without you. You bless my life beyond words with your unwavering love, support, and encouragement.

The entire Thoele, Hall, and Williamson clan, who have so diligently (although sometimes begrudgingly) changed their eating habits. You have shown me that sharing my knowledge and being an example does indeed create positive ripples with wide-reaching effects.

My most faithful, ever-present friends and cheerleaders—Momma Sue, Paige, Jules and Marty—who have spent countless hours over dinners, cocktails, or coffee, listening to my struggles and strife, my wins and worries, and my hopes and dreams for this book. You will never know how each encouraging word was the wind that carried me.

Dr. Scott Vander Wall, Dr. Robert Arne, and Dee Dee Woodman—the extraordinary healers who have helped keep my body, mind, and Spirit optimally functioning during this heart-wrenching process.

My team of pre-publication midwives—Nadège, Gretchen, Stephanie, and Sarah—who helped me finish when my tank was far beyond empty. And a most special thank you to Chelsea, my dear friend and sister, who stood by my side, held my hand, and coached the creative process in the final stages of never-ending labor.

All of my Unseen Helpers who have heard my every request, and guided me, without question, every single day.

My many reinforcement troops—Melinda, Christine and Roger, Tim and Amie, Norm, Fuzzy—and all of the people I've met along the way (you know who you are!)—I thank you from the bottom of my heart for your oh-so-needed boosts of reassurance.

And last but certainly not least, my Beloved fiancé, Brett. Heaven knows that without you, this book would not exist. Thank you for being the *Absolute Best of Everything*. I Love You with All My Heart.

TABLE OF CONTENTS

LIGHTEN *your* TOXIC LOAD®

BOOK ONE

INTRODUCTION:
Who, Why, What, and How?

*"I alone cannot change the world, but I can cast a stone across
the waters to create many ripples."*
—MOTHER TERESA

WHO AM I?

I am a born-and-raised Southern California girl, and perhaps, true to the cliché, my penchant for health, wellness, and everything alternative began there. I suppose the stage was set pretty early in my life, thanks to my mom. Much to my dismay as a child, I was not allowed to eat sugary cereals or drink soda, and I always had a healthy sack lunch for school. Dinner was usually home-cooked from scratch, with only the occasional frozen dinner—usually Stouffer's® Macaroni and Cheese or French Bread Pizza—when my parents worked late or hadn't prepared dinner in advance. But later, in my unruly teenage years, I indulged in my fair share of junk food and unhealthy habits. I consumed Carl's Jr.® hamburgers for lunch, Egg McMuffins® for breakfast, Doritos® for munchies, and… mind-altering substances on the weekends. But all of these unhealthy habits existed right alongside hi-impact aerobics classes (it was the '80s after all), gymnastics training and competition, and occasional trips to the local, what used-to-be, hole-in-the-wall health food café and juice bar that swam in the earthy aromas of brewer's yeast and freshly-grown sunflower sprouts.

With a little prodding from my older and wiser sister, my more inherently-driven health-capades took off just shortly after high school. New habits evolved slowly. My water bottle became a new appendage. I chose to substitute raw vegetables for crunchy snack foods. And then, in my early college days, I opted for a vegetarian diet (but mostly because meat was too expensive for my meager budget). I later read snippets from *Diet for a New America,* by John Robbins, which gave vegetarianism a whole new meaning for me, to say the least. Indeed, his words and images were my very first introduction to the horrors of our Industrial Agriculture system.

Still, I only dabbled until around 1995 when I was attending college at UCLA. That's when my food studies began in earnest, and I wholeheartedly embarked on this passionate life-long-learning-adventure. I read everything I could get my hands on and quickly became quite savvy about the multitude of chemicals and crap in our food. This information rapidly motivated me to shop exclusively at health food stores and co-ops. Lucky for me, I was surrounded by them.

Since then, my life as a whole has been dedicated to optimal health and healing—physically, mentally, emotionally, and spiritually—both personally and professionally. From a master's degree in spiritual psychology, to facilitating hundreds of week-long wild dolphin swims in crystal-clear Bahamian waters, to my own miraculous healing with EMDR therapy, to practicing massage and energy medicine, to teaching (mostly by example) those near and dear to me about healthy eating habits, to a lifelong commitment to growing and evolving. Whew! It goes on and on. My life most definitely revolves around the pursuit of optimal health, true happiness, and well-being.

With that said, it is important to confess that I am far from perfect when it comes to life choices, food or otherwise. Who is? And how boring would *that* be?! Although I am obsessively picky about what I put IN and ON my body, I also adore a rich organic red wine, silky dark chocolate, Red Hot Blues® (the best tortilla chips ever), and mimosas with the rare Sunday brunch. My absolute favorite splurge is super spicy Mexican food combined with the *perfect* margarita— made with fresh lime juice and extra tequila, to satiate my Irish blood. But these big splurges are saved for the occasional night out, when I am really in the mood to blow off some steam and throw caution to the wind. You see, I truly believe life is for living, and that Love, Joy, and Happiness are our true purpose. I also believe that balance is key to a healthy existence, and sometimes that means you just have to savor what you really want!

That's why this series is all about how—and why—to *lighten* your toxic load. Besides, completely *eliminating* toxins is not only next-to-impossible, unless you are "the boy in a bubble," but also virtually unmanageable, if you want to enjoy any kind of social life… at least in our current state of affairs. But learning to choose wisely is vitally important.

WHY AM I WRITING THIS BOOK?

About four years ago, I began researching toxins in cosmetics, thinking that would be my topic for this book. I naïvely thought that toxic food was old news and that most people knew all about the dangers of our industrialized food supply. How wrong I was!

The turning point for me—the catalyst for this book—was the diagnosis of my sister-in-law's breast cancer. It was such a shock to learn that this beautiful, vibrant, young mother—who certainly *looked* healthy—wasn't. Thankfully, after 3½ years of invasive, barbaric treatments, she recovered and is well today. But this eye-opening event also awakened my fire. I began to hear the overwhelming amount of everyday chit-chat about disease and illness and depression and insomnia and prescriptions and suicide and infertility . . . and, and, and. It's like most everyone has succumbed to seeing these issues as normal side-effects of living. Yee Gods! The fact is, there is a great deal of *needless* suffering happening on a very large scale. And I knew that food—and pharmaceuticals—were huge players. I began to vent and complain to my fiancé . . . A LOT. When he sufficiently tired of my grumblings, he finally said, "You either need to stop complaining about all of this or do something about it." So I decided to do something—and you're looking at it.

As I embarked upon this project, I knew that even if it wasn't possible for a person to fully heal too-far-gone health issues, he/she could at least live a much higher quality of life with clean nutrition. I also knew that even if a person appears well today, he/she would be *much* better off in the long run by making healthier choices *now*. Most people need to be hit over the head with some kind of grave crisis to force significant lifestyle changes, but I thought "Maybe, just *maybe* I could help before tragedy had to strike to get someone's full attention?"

That was and is my hope.

"Just because you're not sick doesn't mean you're healthy."
—*AUTHOR UNKNOWN*

TURNS OUT, I DIDN'T KNOW THE HALF OF IT

Until I began the true research process, I only had a vague idea of the reality of our food system. I was already keenly aware of the adulterated and toxic nature of our industrially-produced food, but what I didn't know is how politics and greed determine why all of this sh*# is in our food in the first place, and that's also the reason why people are fed a 5-star buffet of confusing and inaccurate health information. But what really got my goat was the social injustice of it all—the absolute disregard and lack of compassion for humanity, all in the name of money. Allowing people—and the planet—to suffer for the sake of profit is *unthinkable* to me. While at the same time, the government spews all of this talk about the "health care crisis," when the government itself—fueled by Crooked Corporations—sits back and helps create the whole damn thing. I mean, c'mon!

This may seem elementary to many, but what I learned is this: Unchecked Corporate Power—along with government officials for sale—is the crux of all the issues we face in this country. The entire globe actually. As such, I see our food system issues as a *micro of the macro*—a bite-sized picture of what's going awry on the grand scale. And since eating is a necessity, I figure food is the perfect place to begin.

"Few of us are aware that the act of eating can be a powerful statement of commitment to our own well-being, and at the same time the creation of a healthier habitat. Your health, happiness, and the future of life on earth are rarely so much in your own hands as when you sit down to eat."
—JOHN ROBBINS

AND THEN ANGER CAME TO VISIT

As I started to unearth some disturbing realities, I got pretty pissed off. So I knew it would most likely stir anger and contempt in you, too. And rightly so. If we weren't riled up, we'd surely be dead. Or over-medicated. Or distracted by our Smartphone. However, the last thing I want to do is create more anger, negativity, and fear in the world. Because the last thing we need is more of all that. So I found myself confused about how to present what I've learned. I also wondered how in the world these people sleep at night. I sat with my questions and confusion for days, asked for guidance, and here's what came.

The Art of Deception

First, I thought long and hard about my own personal experience with people I've known (and dearly loved) who put profit before people. I came to realize that these experiences were the birth of my great disdain for half-truths, lying, and manipulative behavior. But I also noticed that this experience provided me with some pretty good insight into the inner workings of minds that value money over compassion and integrity. Here's what I learned after listening to countless sales pitches over the years: These people *absolutely,* without a doubt, believed the stories they told. They also dehumanized their customers by using derogatory names and stereotypes, which made it easier to see them as dollar signs instead of human beings. Kinda crazy, but very true. And all the while, these sales-motivated-minds belonged to people who are in fact good-hearted at their core, but consistently made what I considered unscrupulous choices.

Even if the economic scales of a Corporation or a billionaire exist in an entirely different Universe from people I've known, human beings are human beings. As such, I have come to assume that the Corrupt, Controlling Entities must truly believe they aren't doing anything harmful or unjust, at least outwardly. Ruled by materialism, a belief in scarcity (even though filthy rich), and an insatiable appetite for power and control, they have perfected the Art of Rationalization, Justification, Denial, and probably some severe dehumanization, too. And while they may have originally set out to accomplish noble goals, like feeding the world, I think these human beings have simply succumbed to the "dark side," if you will.

"Harder still it has proved to rule the dragon money…
A whole generation adopted false principles and went to their graves in the belief
they were enriching the country they were impoverishing."
—RALPH WALDO EMERSON

Greed as a Mental Illness

And then I watched the movie, *I AM*.

 I AM, THE MOVIE:

This extraordinary documentary—with its many poignant and insightful messages—was exactly what the doctor ordered. If you haven't seen this incredible movie, I highly recommend it! www.Iamthedoc.com The movie, directed by comedy guy Tom Shadyac—perhaps best known for movies such as *Ace Ventura, Bruce Almighty,* and *The Nutty Professor*—"started by asking what's wrong with the world, and ended up discovering what's right with it." What a powerful blast of inspiration!

Not surprisingly, *I AM* talks about greed as the fundamental issue in our world, and how we run the world—and businesses—as a machine, completely disconnected from nature, without any consideration of the future consequences of our actions. Likewise, we treat the economy as a living, breathing entity, while the Earth itself is largely treated like a vending machine. For being relatively intelligent creatures, we sure make some really short-sighted choices, don't ya think?

But here was the biggie for me:

To many native cultures around the globe, greed is a mental illness. The Cree, a Native American tribe, even have an indigenous word for greed. They call it "wétiko," which literally means cannibal: one who eats the life of another for profit.

> [For the wétiko] "Brutality knows no boundaries. Greed knows no limits. Perversion knows no borders. . . . These characteristics all push towards an extreme, always moving forward once the initial infection sets in. . . . This is the disease of the consuming of other creatures' lives and possessions."
> —JACK D. FORBES, "COLUMBUS AND OTHER CANNIBALS: THE WÉTIKO DISEASE OF EXPLOITATION, IMPERIALISM, AND TERRORISM"

This little piece of wisdom really helped me make sense of all the madness I was uncovering. Since, as highlighted in this remarkable movie, human nature is hardwired for love, compassion, and cooperation, I can't think of a more reasonable explanation for how we can possibly hurt members of our own species, animals, or the planet in exchange for riches. Seeing greed as a form of mental illness put things into a whole new perspective for me.

Purposeful Anger

Also, I realized that it is imperative to point out that anger isn't always a negative force. Anger is a basic human emotion that can most definitely serve a constructive purpose, like writing a book! The way I see it, then, is that the very best thing we can do is use anger as motivation—fuel—for positive action.

*"Humanity is going to require a substantially
new way of thinking if it is to survive."*
—ALBERT EINSTEIN

MONEY IS NOT THE PROBLEM...GREED IS

I also want to be sure you understand, I am not anti-money, corporations, or government. But I have absolutely no patience for the actions within these structures that abuse and disrespect humanity.

I am not *at all* against having money, not in the least. Money may not buy happiness or love, but it certainly does provide freedom and options and opportunities. And I'm all about those! Here's the thing: Although money can be a sticky, sticky trap that can completely devour one's focus, it can also be a GREAT tool when used for bringing more Light, Love, Happiness, Compassion, Meaningful Purpose, and Generosity into your life, and thus into the world. In fact, I believe one of the VERY best things we can possibly do in life is to strive to be truly happy and loving. That way, we become a gift to the world simply because we exist. And if money can help nurture these life-enhancing qualities, then by all means! It's the same for government and corporations. Money can most certainly be a great thing.

CHANGE IS UP TO US

As I mention later in this book, and will probably mention repeatedly, WE got ourselves into this mess by not paying attention (and buying into the well-designed distractions). Now it's time to get ourselves out. We need to wake up and take responsibility for ourselves and our planet. We need to accept where we are, move on, and stop expecting the world to change without our efforts. Creating the happy, healthy, peaceful world we all want is up to you and me. Right NOW.

HOW THIS BOOK SERIES IS DESIGNED

The books in this series are specifically designed to be read in order. Each book will build on the previous one, and if you miss a concept, you'll probably be a little lost. This is especially true with this first book, which lays the groundwork for the entire series. Also, each book lays out simple, yet consistent action steps that will gradually move you in the direction of optimal health and well-being, should you choose to take them. So reading the books in order is essential not only for education's sake, but also for your personal success, if your goal is to effectively and permanently lighten your toxic load.

And, when you follow the action steps as the series progresses, I suspect you'll find the lightening process easier than you think. After a short while, you'll most likely begin to crave life-depleting foods *less* and life-supporting foods *more*. Feeling healthy is often a very powerful feedback mechanism, complete with its own set of intrinsic rewards.

WHAT CAN YOU EXPECT TO LEARN?

We will begin with The Politics in this first book, which I see as integral to understanding why it can be so challenging to eat well and to know *what* to eat. And since it is the common thread, The Politics will continue to unfold with each new topic. Furthermore, as we move forward in the series, we will cover everything from Processed Foods to GMOs to Food Packaging to Industrial Agricultural practices to Organics 101 to Advanced Organics to Water to Seafood to Alternative Health Information, Suggestions and Tips, and so, so much more. This series will be your one-stop-shop toward fully understanding each and every aspect of our food system—from the forces of corruption that have kept everything in place to why it is vitally important for you take control of your own health—and of course how. You won't just learn about the issues, you will learn how to become the solution. Before you know it, you will have helped create a happier, healthier world not only for yourself and your family, but for the entire planet, as well as future generations to come.

My website, www.lightenyourtoxicload.com, provides a virtual library of information: references, videos, ways to take action, links to my favorite products and most trusted brands, etc. And it will continue to grow as the series unfolds.

WHAT TYPES OF CHANGES DO I HOPE TO SEE?

- High-quality, healthy, sustainable, chemical-free food for everyone —not just the ones who can currently afford it.

- Unobstructed circulation of accurate, transparent, and truthful information about health and nutrition, allowing us the freedom to *easily* make educated choices that support our well-being.

- Honesty and Integrity within our food system. Compassion and Caring for others, and the Nurturing of our precious planet.

- A highly educated, empowered, critical mass of the American population that is actively involved in our democratic process. Government of the people, by the people, for the people, just as our founding fathers intended.

- And ultimately: Aiming to thrive on local, organic, sustainable foods, grown by farmers we know by name as well as in our own backyards.

From all of my research, this is what I know for sure:

Each one of us would do well to cultivate more independence when it comes to taking care of the basic needs of ourselves, our families, and our communities. Taking our power back and becoming more self-reliant is a necessary goal. And learning where our food comes from, along with what's in it, and why, is the perfect place to begin.

"I believe that the community—in the fullest sense: a place and all its creatures—is the smallest unit of health and that to speak of the health of an isolated individual is a contradiction in terms."
—WENDELL BERRY,
"THE ART OF THE COMMONPLACE: THE AGRARIAN ESSAYS"

These are the goals. And they are BIG. Maybe even utopian. But we gotta start somewhere, right?

IN CLOSING

Writing this book forced me to learn about subjects I previously avoided like the plague—economics, history, and politics—so I by no means claim to be any sort of expert on these matters. However, I have taught myself a tremendous amount by doing massive amounts of research. Consequently, I've been able to take some fairly complex issues, digest them to the best of my ability, and regurgitate the CliffNotes™ version to hopefully give you a relatively clear picture of where we stand. My prose may be imperfect, and my subjects may contain a hole here and there, but I have poured my blood, sweat, and certainly tears into creating the most complete, highly referenced, yet condensed source of information possible.

This project has been a long and arduous road to say the least, and much more challenging than I ever anticipated. Truth be told, had I known what a beast of a project this would be, I would've never started. The stress has made me pretty darn sick at times; I considered quitting on several occasions. And my extraordinary and incredibly supportive fiancé has walked the entire path right alongside me. And there is no way I could be doing this without him. It has not been easy for either of us, but we both know that it's beyond important. I'm hoping that even people who think that what they eat doesn't really matter all that much *will* care about the bigger picture and get involved.

I've had many people tell me that this book will meet a lot of resistance—that most people don't want to know or change. And while sadly that's probably true, I am not writing for those people. I am writing for YOU. Whoever you are, and for whatever reason you are reading, thank you so much. The world needs you.

ARE YOU READY? LET'S DO THIS!

"A small group of thoughtful people could change the world. Indeed, it's the only thing that ever has."
—MARGARET MEAD

CHAPTER 1:
The Dark Age of Health and Nutrition

"The doctor of the future will no longer treat the human frame with drugs, but rather will cure and prevent disease with nutrition."
—THOMAS EDISON

One hundred years from now, I bet we'll refer to this time in history as something like *The Dark Age of Health and Nutrition*. I say this because even with all of our technological "advancements" and modern medicine, people are more chronically ill and more depressed than ever. And when you start digging around in the dirt, the major causes are certainly no mystery.

Truth be told, a very dark, ugly machine is driving the disintegrating health of our world, and it's called Corporate Greed. What does this Machine devour for breakfast, lunch, dinner, and a midnight snack? Platefuls and platefuls of Profit. And its appetite is *insatiable*.

The Corporate "personality" is indeed addicted, obsessed, and possessed. Money, the heartbeat and lifeblood of The Corporation, determines this culture's highly dysfunctional definition of "success." So much so that care and concern for the health and well-being of humanity, animals, and the environment at large is often ignored, justified, or denied.

The reality is that while many people, young and old, are sick and suffering, Corporations are thriving.

Make no mistake about it, chronic illness is Big Business.

So is Food.

And Chemicals.

And unfortunately, they often walk hand-in-hand-in-hand.

CHRONIC DISEASES ARE ON THE RISE

It is becoming increasingly apparent that exposure to environmental toxins is a *major* contributor to the climbing rates of chronic disease. Our bodies are simply carrying too heavy of a toxic load to remain healthy and well.

In fact, the rate of chronic disease has been skyrocketing, and only within the last 35 to 40 years.[1] Take a look at this small sampling of recent trends in the United States:

- Leukemia, brain cancer, and other childhood cancers have shown an overall increase of more than 20% since 1975.[2]

  Specifically, for example, between 1975 and 2004, primary brain cancer increased by nearly 40% while leukemia increased by over 60% among children 14 years and younger.[3]

  Note: Although some statistics can seem hopeful by stating only slight increases in childhood cancer rates—at 0.6% each year since 1975[4]—that statistic is misleading. A 0.6% increase per year, compounded, is equivalent to an *overall increase* of 24% in 36 years.[5] And that's no small potatoes.

- A woman's lifetime risk of breast cancer has increased from 1 in 10 in 1973, to 1 in 8 in 2013.[6-7]

- Asthma prevalence approximately doubled between 1980 and 1995.[8]

  In 2011, nearly 1 in 12 Americans had asthma, and those numbers are increasing every year.[9]

  Note: Asthma and food allergies—which were virtually unheard of 30 years ago—are now appearing inextricably linked. Children who suffer with (true) food allergies are cited as 2 to 4 times more likely to be afflicted with asthma than those without food allergies.[10]

- The incidence of autism spectrum disorders has skyrocketed by nearly 300% between 1997 and 2008.[11]

  In 2000, an estimated 1 in 150 American children had a form of autism. In 2006, 1 in 110. In 2008, 1 in 88.[12] And the most recent 2012 estimate? 1 in 50.[13]

And those concerns are just a piece of the pie. There is also chronic obesity, heart disease, autoimmune issues (such as Type-1 diabetes or celiac disease), neurological disorders (such as Parkinson's or Alzheimer's), digestive disturbances (such as irritable bowel syndrome or acid reflux), and catch-all terms like "chronic fatigue syndrome," all of which are way too common in our daily conversations these days.

SO WHAT'S CHANGED?

We currently live in a world vastly ruled by Big Chemical Corporations. As a result, our "technologically advanced" world is now inundated with various forms of chemical pollution, with the food we eat—the way it's grown, processed, and *created*—being a major contributor to the growing list of common medical issues.

The now widespread practice of using wicked amounts of chemicals in conventional agriculture, along with the far-from-natural ingredients used in processed products, allows the massive industrialization of incredibly cheap food. Using these methods, crops and animals grow larger and faster, and processed food remains edible for eons. This relatively new method of food production is obviously not healthy for you or me, but ridiculously profitable for the Controlling Corporations.

Yes, indeed, Big Chemical Corporations are made filthy rich by polluting our bodies and the planet with toxic chemicals. To add insult to injury, they cash in once more via Big Pharmaceutical-Chemical-Corporations. How? They treat the consequences of toxic overload with prescription drugs and expensive medical treatments.

In a nutshell, Big Chemical Corporations create
the problem and then offer the solution.
Cha-ching! *Cha-ching!*

This machine is a self-perpetuating cash crop.

Although this probably wasn't what Big Chemical Corporations intentionally set out to accomplish, it has most certainly evolved into a brilliant business model, with incredibly seductive results.

THE LINK BETWEEN FOOD AND DECLINING HEALTH

So you might be wondering—what exactly IS in the food we eat, anyway?

For now, suffice it to say, there are literally thousands upon thousands of Food and Drug Administration (FDA)-*approved* (but not necessarily safe) ingredients in our food. The infinite list of items include things like pesticides, herbicides, hormones, antibiotics, various miscellaneous pharmaceuticals, genetically modified organisms (GMOs), and artificial-everything-you-could-ever-imagine, just to name the heavy hitters.

Truth be told, most people are living on lab-created, poison-laden, drug-infused, mass-produced, processed foods. Or, in other words, *processed chemicals disguised as food*. I am not only referring to all of the packaged "foods" on the shelves in the middle aisles of your local supermarket, but to all of the conventionally raised fruits, vegetables, meats, and dairy, too. Nearly all conventionally produced foods are a virtual shell of their former selves. Jam-packed, covered, or smothered with stuff we were simply and utterly never designed to *purposefully* eat.

I can imagine you might be scratching your head right about now and wondering…

BUT THE STUFF WE EAT *IS* SAFE, RIGHT?

As it will become increasingly clear in the following chapters, not the way most people eat, and certainly not for the long haul. Unfortunately, it can be difficult to *prove* that certain chemicals, ingredients, or methods of food production *cause* specific health issues. Why? Chronic diseases related to a toxic diet can often take years to accumulate and manifest (which also means there is time to reverse the damage), so linking the cause of an illness to a specific food or ingredient is riddled with confounding factors.

While science does know—often without advertising—that certain ingredients are in fact toxic to our bodies, others have yet to be *proven* toxic. The FDA ingredient "safety system" is pretty much "innocent until proven guilty." That is, many ingredients are qualified as Generally *(generally???)* Recognized As Safe (GRAS) without proper safety testing. As a consequence, trying to prove the link between illness or death and a specific ingredient is not common practice unless a relatively large group of people get sick or die at the same time—suddenly and mysteriously.

So the answers to important questions about what's in our food are often inconclusive. For example, can the artificial sweetener aspartame *cause* autism? We don't know for sure. In fact, there are at least *10* chemicals suspected to contribute to autism and learning disabilities, six of which can be found in food. And yes, aspartame is one of those listed chemicals. Do genetically modified organisms *cause* gut issues that can lead to other devastating health issues? Again, we don't know for sure. Often, there are other factors involved, such as genetic predisposition, or a combination of toxins in the body that create just the right formula for catastrophe.

The point is, *we don't know*.

And as we will see in chapters to come, while it is typically difficult to prove that specific foods cause illness and disease, *the correlations* between specific toxins and health issues can be so profound, that to ignore them would be unwise. There is also common sense. I mean, c'mon, does it really make sense to eat chemicals that are designed to kill living organisms?

I don't know about you, but I'm not willing to sit around and just wait until the proof is in the pudding. Think *Tobacco*. What did the Tobacco Industry say? "Oh yes! Of course, it's safe, it's safe, it's safe!" Until years and years and years later it turned out that chronic tobacco use was not only unsafe, but absolutely devastating-beyond-imagination to human health.

THE CHEMICAL COCKTAIL

What we do know for certain is that many chemicals in our world are toxic to the body, and toxic overload leads to disease.

Pretty Simple Stuff, Right?

One chemical residue floating around in the body, be it a "residue" of a pesticide, antibiotic, hormone, one of the thousands of artificial ingredients, or a GMO, is most likely easily handled by our bodies. But tally up all of the "residues" found in our environment to which we are exposed on a daily basis, and we've got a lot to manage. In fact, all of those itty, bitty amounts of tolerable toxins can combine in unknown ways to create a "chemical cocktail."

Chemistry 101

Chemicals create reactions when combined. One relatively benign chemical can become volatile and toxic when mixed with another. Many of us have an image, or perhaps a personal memory, etched in our minds of chemistry class and the spontaneously-exploding-beaker. The explosion, of course, is a consequence of an inaccurate combination of chemicals. You can think of your body as that beaker in chemistry class.

The reality is that we simply have no clue what happens in the body when it's exposed to a mishmash of multiple chemicals. And frankly, there is absolutely no way to test the infinite combinations of chemicals that might occur inside of us. And, as we are learning, our food, water, prescription drugs, and entire environment is saturated with abundant known *and unknown* chemicals.

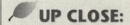 **UP CLOSE:**

"A study at Tufts University by Ann Soto tested the effect of 10 pesticides which mimic estrogen in the body. At low levels, one pesticide alone had virtually no effect on the human body. However, when combined, various pesticides showed strong estrogen-mimicking effects even at low levels."[14]

IT'S NOT JUST OUR FOOD THAT'S TOXIC

Nearly every conventional cosmetic product (from shampoo to toothpaste, lotion to shaving cream, mascara to aftershave) and household cleaner is also full of synthetic, harmful chemical ingredients. Then add items more difficult or nearly impossible to avoid (or readily change) such as household furnishings, building materials, and our outdoor air quality. We inhale these chemicals into our lungs, and we absorb them through our skin. All of these various residues contribute to the chemical cocktail and our overall toxic load.

And then there is our tap water. What you may not realize is that all of the various chemical contaminants that we use every day eventually find their way back into our tap water, which means we are now drinking all of these chemicals, too. Our tap water—even bottled in many cases—is brimming with chemicals so abundant that many are not yet even classified.

> ### 🍃 DID YOU KNOW?
>
> More than 80,000 new synthetic chemicals have been created since World War II. These chemicals are now utilized in millions of products, from foods to cleaning products to cosmetics to clothing, building materials, children's toys, and baby bottles.[15,16]

IS EVERYONE GOING TO GET SICK? OF COURSE NOT!

We've all heard about the 105-year-old man who chain-smoked cigars and drank a pint of Jack Daniel's every single day of his life but was healthy as a horse until his very last breath. As you might imagine, I get this argument from people all the time.

Do you know if you are one of those super-power-people? Nope. Neither do I. Some people are simply more susceptible to disease and illness than others. Furthermore, the quality of our food, water, and the health of our environment is not what it used to be. I am amazed at the good health of many of my elders, but then I remember that they had a solid foundation as youngsters. They actually ate clean, unadulterated food for most of their lives, like corn-on-the-cob straight out of their backyard garden, or milk and eggs fresh from their very own farm. These amazing elders are also very happy, engaged with life and their community, while continuing to take great care of their bodies, minds, and spirits to this day. And all of those factors play into their good health.

People are indeed living longer as a whole, but how many of the elderly are as healthy as the ones I know? According to the U.S. National Center for Health Statistics, 45% of American adults 65 and older now suffer from *two or more* chronic conditions. That means that almost half of the elderly population is not well, and that number has been steadily increasing over the last decade.[17]

Is living a longer life worth the price of suffering in poor health, dependent upon pharmaceutical drugs? Not in my book. Not even for a second. But I can hardly bear feeling miserable with a cold for a week!

One thing I know for sure, I can help myself stay as healthy as possible by significantly reducing my toxic load. You can, too!

THE *BOTTOM* LINE

- *The Dark Age of Health and Nutrition = The Golden Age of Prosperity* for Controlling Corporations and Big Industry.

- We live in a chemical world and it's up to YOU to take responsibility for your health.

THE REALLY GOOD NEWS!

There are many toxins in your world that you cannot control, but food and water are not among them! You have absolute power when it comes to choosing what you eat and what you drink.

And the really, really good news?!

Your body is *miraculously resilient* when given the proper nutrition to thrive. That means whatever potential harm has been done can also be undone! If you provide the foundation for good health with nutrient-dense food, clean water, exercise, and regular detoxification, your body has the ability to sufficiently metabolize and release a substantial amount of toxic deluge.

WHAT YOU CAN DO RIGHT NOW

If you'd like to get a jump-start on the process of Lightening Your Toxic Load, drink purified water. Here are a few options:

- Purchase a water filter. Even a simple Brita or PUR pitcher (or something similar) is better than tap water. If it's in your budget, you can purchase an under-the-counter or countertop system, but please make sure to do your research before making a choice. Some systems filter more contaminants than others, and they can be pricey.

- Sign up for bottled spring water home delivery. You can go to www.findaspring.com to find a source near you. As stated on their site, "Please independently test all spring water before you make the decision to consume it." Spring water is not always as pure as we'd like to believe!

- Use the water filter machines often located at your local supermarket or natural food store. They can also sometimes be found outside gas stations or convenience stores. Make sure to check the service date on the machine so you can ensure the filter system is optimally functioning.

NOTE: I'll be providing much more information on water and the best filtration options later in this series.

NEXT CHAPTER

We'll take a detailed look at the hard truth surrounding the *Politics of Food.* You will learn about the tactics used by Controlling Corporations/Big Industry to keep you in the dark, how they keep our government working for their interests, and why it is vitally important for you to take responsibility for your own health.

"You see there is no money in healthy people, and there is no money in dead people.
The money is in the middle, people who are alive—sort of—
but have one or more chronic conditions."
—BILL MAHER

CHAPTER 2:
The Politics of Food

"The liberty of a democracy is not safe if the people tolerate the growth of private power to the point where it becomes stronger than their democratic state itself. That is, in its essence, fascism..."
—FRANKLIN DELANO ROOSEVELT,
SPEAKING TO THE U.S. CONGRESS, 1938

A CRUCIAL CONSIDERATION

As we begin to lift the veil of secrecy, I would like to offer some words of wisdom from my own personal experience…

If you get caught up in the negativity and the *ain't-they/it-awful* mindset, you'll just become part of the problem. I say this with great understanding. Believe me, I've been there.

I'm not saying you won't be angry. I certainly was! I'm just saying it is best not to get stuck in that space. Transforming anger—a very powerful, action-oriented force—into choices that support the positive advancement of humanity and the environment is an incredibly healthy, functional way to channel all of that energy.

FOOD FOR THOUGHT:

A Cherokee Legend[1]

An old Cherokee is teaching his grandson about life. "A fight is going on inside me," he said to the boy.

"It is a terrible fight and it is between two wolves. One is evil—he is anger, envy, sorrow, regret, greed, arrogance, self-pity, guilt, resentment, inferiority, lies, false pride, superiority, and ego." He continued, "The other is good—he is joy, peace, love, hope, serenity, humility, kindness, benevolence, empathy, generosity, truth, compassion, and faith. The same fight is going on inside you—and inside every other person, too."

The grandson thought about it for a minute and then asked his grandfather, "Which wolf will win?"

The old Cherokee simply replied, "The one you feed."

A WORD TO THE WISE

Please read this chapter slowly. It contains A LOT of information. So, in order to avoid feeling overwhelmed, I highly encourage you to read this chapter in digestible chunks.

KNOWLEDGE IS POWER

From this moment forward, as we take a look at the hard realities that require drastic and immediate action, please remember to keep in mind that **the information I share is not intended to instill fear**. On the contrary, my intention is to help raise awareness and create an attitude of empowerment through education and simple solutions. WE got ourselves into this mess, and now it's time to dig our way out.

So let's get on with it!

THE HARD REALITY

There are billions *upon billions* of dollars generated in the Big Industries of agriculture, pharmaceuticals, food, and chemicals. And these Big Industries are wholeheartedly invested in keeping things just the way they are, even if that means the devastation of public health and the poisoning of our planet. This is a harsh statement, but it's absolutely true.

Plainly stated, our system is corrupt and broken. Corporations—whether privately or publicly held—are infinitely powerful entities that have the ability to possess and control our Government like puppets on a string. Although created to serve and protect the public, our Government and its agencies (such as the FDA and EPA) are mainly serving Corporate Greed.

OUR JACKED-UP SYSTEM

As we will learn shortly, the reality of our artificial, man-made, adulterated food system is meticulously hidden and buried. This is no accident.

Our right to know what's in the things we consume every day—and our freedom to choose—is lost in a sea of manipulated research, deceptive marketing, misleading headlines, ghostwritten articles, label lies, false claims…yadda, yadda, and more yadda.

For the average newspaper reader, Internet surfer, or nightly news watcher, these purposefully designed tactics can make eating—and living—healthfully a confusing and overwhelming undertaking. Exactly as intended.

THE BIG BUSINESS OF FOOD: AGRICULTURE, CHEMICAL, AND PHARMACEUTICAL

Regardless of the illusory images displayed in marketing propaganda, our conventional food system no longer relies on small, independent farmers that cultivate diverse crops by hand, or lovingly raise livestock on pastoral farms. Our conventional food system is now an *Industrialized Entity*, run and controlled by Big Agriculture (Big Ag), Big Chemical (Big Chem), Big Pharmaceutical (Big Pharma), and Big Food.

These Industries are the "people" who now command how our food is grown, raised, medicated, manufactured, and processed. They are also in charge of how our food is marketed, sold, and labeled.

As we will discover shortly, the Big Corporations that make up these massive Industries are impressively savvy at shaping policy to assure their agendas—and their bottom lines—are met.

First, let's get clear on which-Industries-control-what within our food system.

Big Ag:

Grows, produces, and processes our food. They saturate our crops with chemicals and inject our animals with pharmaceuticals so that they can sell cheaper food… faster.

Agriculture behemoth *Cargill* is an example of a Big Ag Corporation. *Forbes* named Cargill the #1 largest private company in America in 2013,[2] cashing in at a whopping $136.7 *billion* in revenue. This is nothing new. Cargill has been #1 on the *Forbes* list for six consecutive years now.

Big Chem:

Manufactures the chemicals that Big Ag sprays on our food. Big Chem—which includes "The Biotech Industry"—also creates the genetically engineered (aka GE, GMO, or GM) seeds and "franken-foods" now rampant in our food system.

As we will see, Genetically Modified crops have created the need for an even greater amount of Big Chem products, in the form of stronger and even more toxic pesticides and herbicides.

The "Big Six" Chemical Corporations that control the world's seed, pesticide, herbicide, and biotechnology industries include *BASF, Bayer, Dow, DuPont, Monsanto,* and *Syngenta.*

Big Pharma:

Keeps our confined and sickly livestock "healthy" and growing at unnaturally rapid rates by providing drugs, like hormones and antibiotics. Big Pharma also cashes in when *we* get sick and "need" drugs from eating all of this incredibly toxic and nutrient-deficient food.

Examples of the Big Pharmaceutical Corporations include *Pfizer, Novarits, GlaxoSmithKline,* and *Merk & Co.*

It's important to note that Big Pharma and Big Chem are inextricably linked. As you probably recognize, most of the Big Six Chemical Corporations listed above are also involved in pharmaceuticals, to varying degrees. Pharmaceuticals, after all, are most often created from synthetic chemicals.

Big Food:

Manufactures, labels, markets, and sells processed "food." These Corporations are largely responsible for the creation—and addictive nature—of junk foods. With their deplorable products and gargantuan marketing budgets, Big Food supports and applauds ever-declining nutrition standards.

Some examples of The Big Food Corporations include *Coca-Cola, General Mills, ConAgra,* and *Kraft.*

And by the way, the diversity of brands you see on supermarket shelves is just an illusion. Only a handful of these large Corporations own them *all*.

THE BOTTOM LINE

Our industrialized food system is not about quality food or optimal health. It's about selling cheap, addictive food as-quickly-as-chemically-possible.

BIG AG, BIG CHEM, BIG PHARMA, AND BIG FOOD ARE ALL PITCHING FOR THE SAME TEAM.

These Industries—and the Corporations within—all benefit from a mutually supportive relationship—keeping one another fat and happy.

Together, these Industries decide what goes into and on our food... and how much we are allowed to know.

HOW DO THESE BIG BUSINESSES ASSURE THEIR AGENDAS ARE MET?

Primary tool? Heaps and loads and tons of Big Money, of course!

As you may or may not know, Corporations use extensive economic resources to influence policy outcomes, "scientific" research, and YOUR perspective.

By providing financial incentives such as boosting research budgets for universities, allocating bonus compensation for scientists, awarding speaking fees, giving generous and well-thought-out gifts, sponsorships, royalty payments, dividends, job promotions, and proceeds from the sale of start-up companies—you probably get the picture—Corporations can always recruit far-reaching help to support their success.

Whether they are scientists-for-hire, researchers at academic universities, the FDA, journalists, or members of Congress—simply put—human beings are vulnerable to the power of economic enticement.

Now, let's dive in and take a detailed look at how Corporations (and Industry at large) use money and power to persuade the world around them to produce whatever is necessary to accomplish their goals.

CORPORATE/INDUSTRY-SPONSORED RESEARCH

Corporate/Industry-Sponsored Research

The first vitally-important thing for you to know is that many "safety studies"—the ones conducted to prove that food ingredients, drugs, or chemicals are safe for human consumption—are often *directly paid for by the Corporation* that created the product. Let's see how this works.

When sponsoring their own research, Corporations have several custom-tailored options from which to choose when conducting a study.

They can opt to:

- Do their studies in-house.

- Hire private scientists.

- Hire academic universities.

- Provide funding for non-profit organizations such as the American Diabetes Association.

- Hire private, nonacademic, for-profit research groups—known as contract research organizations (CROs).

The thing is, when Corporations sponsor their own research, they apparently also reserve the right to make their own rules.

Specifically, they can:

- Reserve the right to pre-publication review, which allows them to publish studies that show *only* desirable results.[3]

- Withhold, manipulate, or delay the content of research results.[4,5]

- Conceal conflicts of interest, including financial agreements or biased relationships, with those conducting the Corporation's research.[6]

- Restrict their researchers from contributing to the trial design, accessing the raw data, interpreting the results, or independently publishing results/making results known to the public.[6,7]

If you know the slightest bit about scientific method, then you know that these allowances in research are insane. And if you don't know squat about scientific method, I am here to tell you that making these allowances in research is insane! When the results of important safety studies can literally be bought, buried, or manipulated—that would be called something like *crooked capitalism*—not research.

SIMPLY PUT: When Corporations fund their own research, they can also create their own rules. Among other things, this gives Corporations the capacity to exert power over the people who are directly involved with the approval of their products.

Which, of course, begs the question:

Can we really trust the results of studies that are funded and controlled by the very Corporations who stand to profit from those results?

It is definitely a good question, and one being asked by honest and concerned researchers around the world. And, not too surprisingly, abundant reviews do indeed document the fact that study results are often biased in favor of the sponsoring Corporation, showing significant associations between Industry funding and pro-Industry conclusions.[6]

For instance:

- A review of studies on the chemicals alachlor, atrazine, formaldehyde, and perchloroethylene found that 60% of studies conducted by independent (non-industry) researchers reported these substances to be hazardous chemicals, while only 14% of Industry-sponsored studies came to the same conclusion.[8]

- A study of review articles on the health effects of secondhand smoke from tobacco found that 74% of those who denied the harmful health effects of secondhand tobacco smoke had connections to the Tobacco Industry.[9]

- Nutrition research sponsored by the Food Industry is more likely to end up favoring the food under consideration than independently-funded research.[10]

Even doctors receive economic incentives that, in turn, support Industry:

- Pharmaceutical Industry studies reveal that physicians who receive gifts, travel expenses, meals, or attend Industry-sponsored conferences are more likely to prescribe the sponsor's medications.[11]

In light of conclusions such as these, answering the question of whether we can trust study results to be reported freely, accurately, and legitimately—when scientific integrity can be compromised in exchange for money, gifts, or promotions—sure seems quite obvious.

UP CLOSE:

Gone are the days when the sole purpose of research was the pursuit of knowledge—simply for the sake of gaining knowledge—true, accurate information that guided public health, prosperity, and security.

In the past, we relied largely on academic institutions funded by government grants to fuel knowledge, based on authentic scientific inquiry and integrity. But as Corporations expanded in the 20th century, so did the realization that investing in research could provide a competitive edge. As a consequence, research funding began to shift from the public sector to Private Industry.

Now, according to a 2012 analysis in *The New Atlantis: A Journal of Technology and Society*, approximately 62% of domestic research and development in scientific fields, such as the Chemical or Pharmaceutical Industries, is in fact carried out by Private Industry itself.[12]

This percentage is compared to the federal government, which only funds about 31% of research and development, coming in a far second behind Private Industry. And interestingly—or unfathomably, depending upon who you are—the majority of that government funding is dedicated to research and development of *military weapons*. Ugh.

Corporate Cash and University Research

Many Big Ag and Big Food Corporations support universities with substantial financial contributions. They may provide direct funding, in the case of land-grant universities, or they might make other generous donations such as lab sponsorships, building construction, faculty endowments, or student fellowships. This funding can benefit Corporations in several ways.[13]

For example, in exchange for large donations, a wing of a new building will often display the name of the sponsoring Corporation. For example, Cargill donated $10 million to the University of Minnesota, and voila! The *Cargill Plant Genomics Building* was born.[13] This gives the Corporation a direct presence—a daily advertisement, really—while also promoting good will *and loyalty* between faculty and students.

Furthermore, many land-grant universities now rely quite heavily on Corporate funding for their agricultural research departments and program budgets. For instance, between 2006 and 2010, Iowa State University's agronomy (the science of crop production and soil management) department received research grants totaling $19.5 million—almost half of the department's grant funding—from Private Industry patrons, including the Iowa Soybean Association, Monsanto, and Dow.[14]

Relying on Corporate/Industry funding can, at the very least, discourage independent research. At worst, Corporate funding may allow the Corporation to sway the curriculum or directly influence research programs to suit their own agendas.[13]

Too Close For Comfort

Although there are potential benefits to the merging of Industry and the research community, such as boosting research budgets and opportunities, increasing salaries for researchers, and collaborating on the development of new medicine and treatments, by now you'll probably agree, there is no denying the inherent conflict of interest this marriage presents.

The gosh-darn reality is simply this: Financial relationships can blur the lines between right and wrong when it comes to the duty to uphold the principles of sound science, integrity, and moral obligation. Period.

And, as numerous studies show, financial relationships among Industry and the research community are indeed pervasive.

For example:

- *The Journal of the American Medical Association* conducted a national survey of medical school department heads and found that 60% of the respondents reported a personal relationship with Industry. The authors concluded, "Overall, institutional academic–industry relationships are highly prevalent and underscore the need for their active disclosure and management."[15]

- *The Association of University Technology Managers* reported that 68% of academic research institutions in the United States and Canada held equity in businesses sponsoring research at their respective institutions.[16]

- The *American Journal of Clinical Nutrition* named 28 food and drug companies as sustaining sponsors of their publication, including companies such as Coca-Cola, Gerber, Nestle/Carnation, Monsanto, Procter & Gamble, Slim-Fast Foods, and The Sugar Association.[17]

The examples go on and on… and on.

THE BOTTOM LINE

Corporations can (and do) assure that their manufactured goods are approved for sale—and remain selling—whether they are proven safe or otherwise, by sponsoring their own research, creating their own rules, and supporting the research community in general.

Next, let's take a detailed look at another wily tool that Corporations exploit to help shape—or confuse—public perspective in order to sell their wares…

CORPORATE-SPONSORED INFORMATION: EDITORIALS, ARTICLES, AND VIDEOS

Corporate-Sponsored Information

When Corporations feel threatened or need to boost consumer support, they can hire scientists, doctors, or other subject-appropriate experts to disrupt sound science or contradict existing scientific opinion. These "experts-for-hire" are paid—or compensated in some manner—to write pro-Industry articles or editorials for peer-reviewed journals, highly accredited universities, respected newspapers, periodicals, or even Industry-sponsored websites and videos.

For example:

- The Tobacco Industry invested $156,000 to hire over a dozen scientists to write editorials discrediting a 1993 federal report that connected secondhand smoke to lung cancer. This pro-Industry propaganda was featured in highly accredited journals and periodicals such as the *Journal of Regulatory Toxicology and Pharmacology*, the *Journal of the National Cancer Institute*, the *Journal of the American Medical Association*, *Risk Analysis*, and *The Wall Street Journal*.[18]

- Circa 1997, Wyeth-Ayerst Pharmaceuticals (now Pfizer) hired DesignWrite, an expert-filled marketing firm,[19] to promote public acceptance of the safety and benefits of hormone replacement therapy (HRT) drugs such as Prempro and Premarin.

  Thanks to the University of California at San Francisco's extensive *Drug Document Archive*,[20] we are given a glimpse into truth-telling documents that reveal the depth of deception that can take place behind closed doors. According to UCSF's archive, DesignWrite planted somewhere around 50 reviews and editorials in respected medical journals to support Wyeth's success with HRT drugs. Wyeth-sponsored, DesignWrite-published-papers can be found in respected medical journals such as *Journal of Women's Health, Archives of Internal Medicine, American Journal of Obstetrics and Gynecology,* and *International Journal of Fertility*, among others.[21]

  Just about everything you need to know about Corporate-

Sponsored Information can be clearly traced through Design-Write's extensive business/publication plans for Wyeth.[22,23] These plans spell out key issues and message strategies, primary audiences, targeted peer-reviewed journals, and even financial cost to Wyeth. You can also see examples of company reports,[24] meeting agendas,[25] meeting minutes,[26] and financial invoices[27] that track progress after Wyeth hired DesignWrite.

I encourage you to review these damning documents for yourself. There is a massive amount of information on UCSF's database (http://dida.library.ucsf.edu/), but you can find all of the documents I've cited at my website, www.lightenyourtoxicload.com.

This kind of Corporate information often only becomes available to the public as a result of a lawsuit or investigation. That's what happened here. Many of these previously-confidential documents—as stated on actual documents—are now public information due to the loads of lawsuits associating Wyeth's Prempro with breast cancer.[28]

As I looked at all of this information, I was dumbstruck. It made me wonder how much crucial decision-making information is confidential and hidden from public knowledge *right now*? My guess is A LOT. Probably more than we could ever imagine. Because just as we've seen here, grand master plans are often concealed and protected from public eyes until a Corporation finds itself in a pot of scalding water.

🍃 DID YOU KNOW?

In 2002, results from a Women's Health Initiative study concluded that estrogen plus progestin drugs, such as Prempro, increased the risk of invasive breast cancer.[29] The study also showed an increased likelihood that cancer would advance more quickly when using Prempro. But this information didn't seem to matter much.

Even with the very real threat of increased breast cancer risk, and all of the lawsuits to prove it, Prempro is still on the market. With that said, Prempro does seem to work for some women, side-effect free, as seen in online reviews.[30] However, it clearly doesn't work that way for all, maybe not even most. So, is it really worth the risk?

And besides, should anything with this type of substantial risk be allowed on the market *in the first place*? Should anything *ever* be legally advertised as safe unless the creating Corporation and the FDA are not 200% sure a product is, in fact, SAFE?

The Chicken or the Egg?

Here is one more example of Corporate-Sponsored Information, but it's a curious case. Is Corporate funding the chicken or the egg? It's hard to say. Regardless, this group seems to be hard at work in an effort to shape your perspective. And that seems puurrrty important, so let's take a look...

The pro-Industry group **The American Council on Science and Health (ACSH)**—with the tag line *Science. Not Hype*—claims to be a consumer education and advocacy group relying on peer-reviewed science to dispel myths and fear-mongering in "junk science."

The glut of pro-Industry publications on ACSH's website is so extensive it's crazy, defending every potentially hazardous human and environmental toxin imaginable.[31] ACSH could care less if the EPA has already categorized a substance as carcinogenic or neurotoxic; they still claim nearly anything is absolutely safe to inhale, swallow, or slather on your skin! Oh, except tobacco. Apparently enough people have died from tobacco use to admit that it's a deadly substance.

In addition to their website, ACSH-authored-articles can be found in periodicals such as *Forbes, The New York Post,* and *USA Today*, among many others. ACSH council representatives also appear regularly on TV, radio shows, and in public debates, spewing all kinds of Industry-supportive information.

Here's the curious part. At ACSH's inception in 1978, they were an independent organization that denied any Corporate funding.[32] And from the very beginning, ACSH founders' goal was to refute what they perceived as unsound science, specifically with regard to health and environmental issues that promoted public confusion. This original goal, along with ACSH's intention to remain independent and credible, sure makes it seem like this rather large organization TRULY believes, and always has, that hazardous chemicals are harmless.

However, ACSH began to accept Corporate funding at some point. In fact, from 1984 to 1985, their list of Corporate funders read like an invitation to a lavish Big Industry Ball.[33] Then, shortly thereafter, ACSH stopped publishing information on Corporate Sponsors, probably in an effort to retain credibility.

However, recent financial documents[34] leaked to *Mother Jones* "show that ACSH depends heavily on funding from corporations that have a financial stake in the scientific debates it aims to shape."[35] Once again, these documents show another red-carpet list of Corporate Sponsors running the gamut from Big Food to Big Chem to Big Pharma to Big Ag and even Big Oil. It's the whole enchilada plus a mountain of guacamole!

So the question is: Does ACSH receive Corporate funding to support their own views and further their own agenda? Or does Corporate funding shape their views and agenda? Hard to say, but this is what we know for sure: ACSH is definitely Pro-Industry and Pro-Toxic-Chemicals.

NON-PROFIT HEALTH ORGANIZATIONS: CAN WE TRUST *THEM* TO PROVIDE ACCURATE INFORMATION ABOUT OUR HEALTH?

Not always. Many non-profit organizations receive Corporate funding. For instance, the **American Diabetes Association** has received funding from some of the largest pharmaceutical companies, such as Bayer and Merk & Co., as well as manufacturers of junk food, like General Mills and Kraft.[36]

Another example is **The American Dietetic Association** (now called the Academy of Nutrition and Dietetics—AND for short), which represents and oversees registered dieticians, but is at least partially sustained by Corporate money.

The ADA's (now AND) Corporate-Sponsored "Nutrition Fact Sheets" show that dietary advice can definitely be muddled with food company marketing. You can see examples of "Topics, sponsors, and representative statements in nutrition fact sheets issued by the American Dietetic Association" in a commentary by Marion Nestle,[17] which you can find at www.lightenyour toxicload.com. Suffice it to say that these nutrition "fact" sheets are carefully crafted messages designed to convince you that whatever the sponsoring Corporation is trying to sell is safe and healthy, or at least innocuous.

Furthermore, according to a recent 51-page report by *Eat Drink Politics,* "in 2001, AND listed 10 food industry sponsors; the 2011 annual report lists 38, a more than three-fold increase."[37]

To see a very long list of non-profits that receive Corporate funding, you can go to: www.cspinet.org/integrity/nonprofits/index.html

Lack of Disclosure is the Big Blind

To make matters even more opaque, the authors and orators of pro-Industry propaganda, in the majority of instances, are not required to disclose their financial relationship with the sponsoring Corporation. Especially if they run their own show, as is the case with ACSH.

Although some peer-reviewed journals *intend* to be proactive in managing conflicts of interest with stated "disclosure policies," studies reveal that either very few articles actually do contain financial conflict disclosures, or journals have a malleable definition of what providing disclosure actually means.[38,39]

In fact:

- Research indicates that very few editors of scientific journals require the author to disclose conflicts of interest. Furthermore, 66% of articles found in journals that DO have disclosure policies revealed zero disclosure of financial conflict of interests.[40]

- Do you remember the highly publicized Stanford study claiming that organic food is no more nutritious than conventional? As the *Cornucopia Institute* states: "Stanford researchers claimed independence by stating they had not received outside financial support for their study, but failed to delineate the close ties between their internal funding sources and industrialized agriculture and biotechnology interests."[41]

  The Stanford Study is a particularly interesting example of secretive Corporate sponsorship, which we will explore more deeply later in this book series.

- The *American Journal of Clinical Nutrition* inserts the letter 's' on the page numbers of an Industry-sponsored article, hoping to alert educated readers that the article may have skipped the scrutiny of the peer-review process. [17]

But how many laypeople would possibly know the meaning of that obscure scrap of information? I sure didn't!

📎 DID YOU KNOW?

Not surprisingly, scientific fraud has become much too common.

According to a review of biomedical and life-science research papers published in *Proceedings of the National Academy of Sciences October 1, 2012*: "Incomplete, uninformative or misleading retraction announcements have led to a previous underestimation of the role of fraud in the ongoing retraction epidemic. The percentage of scientific articles retracted because of fraud has *increased ~10-fold since 1975*."[42]

A study might be retracted because the author, editor, or institution can't shake a guilty conscience after publishing inaccurate information in service to Corporate Sponsors, simply for some extra cash. Or maybe, accurate information was published that threatened Corporate profit, and some form of harassment or threat was used to force a retraction.

Whatever the case, increased retraction rates are most likely a symptom of growing Corporate control. One thing we know for sure: Objectivity and neutrality can be compromised when Corporate Cash is King.

THE BOTTOM LINE

Unless you can be sure there are no financial ties or biased relationships that may nurture a conflict of interest, you would be wise to read, watch, and listen to circulating information—whether on the news, in a scientific journal, or published by a highly respected university—with caution and skepticism. Although we are taught to trust expert knowledge, unfortunately, their information can sometimes be misleading at best and fraudulent at worst.

FRONT GROUPS

Corporate-Sponsored Information   Front Groups

According to *SourceWatch*, a front group is defined as "an organization that purports to represent one agenda while in reality it serves some other interest whose sponsorship is hidden or rarely mentioned—typically, a corporate or government sponsor."[43] Front groups might be created by Lobbyists (we'll get to them in the next section), Public Relations Companies, Marketing Firms, or an Industry itself, but regardless of who creates a front group, they are almost always funded by Corporate/Industry interests.

Big Pharma, Big Ag, Big Chem, the Tobacco Industry, Big Food, and most recently the BioTech Industry, all use front groups to convince a skeptical audience to buy their product. Front groups act as a mouthpiece for views that serve their sponsor's economic interests (and thus their own), knowing full well that the educated public will reject the message if they know the sponsor has a vested interest in the message.

Front groups—another, but much larger and more in-depth channel of Corporate-Sponsored Information—also use credentialed spokespeople, such as PhDs and experts in specific fields, to sell their message. They often use smear campaigns and psuedoscience to delude, confuse, and even outwardly lie to the public. As you will see, front groups like to use words like *alliance, coalition, freedom,* and *truth* in the name of their organization, which can be immediately—and purposefully—confusing!

In her acclaimed book, *Diet for a Hot Planet*, Anna Lappé reveals how the Food Industry learned its strategies from Big Tobacco. She quotes a 1969 Tobacco Industry internal memo that reads:

"Doubt is our product. It is the best means of competing with the 'body of fact' that exists in the minds of the general public. It is also the means of establishing a controversy."[44]

Because they are such an incredibly pervasive and effective means for shaping public perspective, I have included several different examples of front groups. Believe it or not, these are just a handful of the *bazillions* of front groups floating around.

Alliance for Food and Farming (AFF)

WWW.FOODANDFARMING.INFO

AFF is an aggressive Agribusiness lobby front group representing the interests of the California Conventional Produce Industry.

As shown by their 2011 California Tax Return,[45] AFF receives substantial financial support from factions of the California Conventional Produce Industry, such as the *California Strawberry Commission* and *California Grape and Tree Fruit*. Many AFF Board Members hold high employment positions within these same Industry groups as well. For instance, the President of the *California Strawberry Commission* is also the Vice Chairman of AFF.[46] The California Conventional Produce Industry relies quite heavily on pesticides to grow their crops,[47] and AFF's job is to help keep it that way.

Toward that end, in July 2010, AFF launched a vigorous campaign attacking the *Environmental Working Group*'s (EWG) "dirty dozen report," which provides consumers with annually-updated information on pesticide residues found on conventionally grown produce.[48] As part of the campaign, AFF created the ostensibly trustworthy site www.safefruitsandveggies.com, in an effort to contest the scientific studies that link synthetic pesticide residues to various health issues.[49] When I checked to make sure this site was still active, it was not only up and running, it was revamped, reenergized... and stomach-turning. This snazzy site is swirling with carefully chosen images, "expert" videos, and sly slogans such as "Moms Deserve the Truth" and "Use Facts, Not Fear, to Make Healthy Food Choices."

AFF's main message: Don't mind the pesticides; just eat your fruit and vegetables!

Clearly, this front group is hell bent on convincing YOU that eating pesticides is A-Okay. And while I wholeheartedly agree that everyone would greatly benefit from eating a lot more fruits and vegetables, it would be *even better* if people could skip the deluge of avoidable poison that often accompanies the conventionally grown varieties. Not rocket science, right?

And don't be fooled— AFF, and many of its sponsors, now claim to support organic agriculture. Seriously???! Since organic methods are the very thing that AFF rallies against, I'm guessing they simply figured this pro-organic illusion would help make them appear less biased and thus, more credible.

We will have a detailed discussion about pesticides in Book Two of this series, as well as a little more about AFF's slippery tactics. For now, I will take this moment to remind you that when you hear the "residue" argument, which is repeatedly used with regard to controversial consumables, remember the "Chemical Cocktail" and your beaker-body!

U.S. Farmers and Ranchers Alliance (USFRA)

WWW.FOODDIAGOGUES.INFO

USFRA is a front group that was formed in response to negative publicity surrounding topics like GMOs and animal welfare. USFRA has a very large "Affiliates, Board Participants, and Industry Partners" list that reads like another red-carpet-who's-who of Big-Ag-Chem-Food, such as Monsanto, DuPont, and loads of conventional meat pushers.[50]

Again, the information and images on this site are skillfully crafted to appalling perfection. It's just a bunch of blah, blah, blah lip service portraying Industrial Ag and all of its unsustainable, toxic practices in a positive, sustainable light, while also attempting to feign a modicum of support for organic agriculture.[51] This seems to be a fashionable trend these days.

You will be learning about every subject covered on this site—from food safety to animal welfare—in depth, as this series progresses. For now, rest assured, trusting information coming from Industry Giants is simply not wise.

Craving more information? Here is an interesting article about USFRA: www.civileats.com/2011/10/05/the-harder-they-spin-what-usfra-wants-us-to-believe-and-why-it's-still-not-the-truth/

While some front groups can be somewhat easily traced for the true source of the message, others are a little more subtle. For example:

Truth in Food

WWW.TRUTHINFOOD.COM

This is a mysterious front group that also hides behind loads of pro-Industrial-Ag propaganda, which is enough to at least question the source of information found on this site. And, with a little poking around, I discovered that this website is maintained by Food-Chain Communications,[52] a marketing firm that specializes in promoting Industrial Agriculture and processed foods.[53] The Truth in Food logo and link is even proudly displayed all over Food-Chain Communications website.

In addition, Food-Chain Communication's founder, Kevin Murphy, has copious connections to many Industrially-proud organizations, including Big Ag beef, dairy, grain, and feed, which are not organizations typically concerned about truth in food, to say the least.[54]

Although the exact message sponsor of the Truth in Food website is not clear, the agenda most certainly is. Industry-specific marketing firms don't just magically appear; they are hired!

CommonGround

WWW.FINDOURCOMMONGROUND.COM

CommonGround is another Big Ag front group brought to you, at least in part, by the United Soybean Board and National Corn Growers Association.[55,56] CommonGround claims to be a grassroots organization run by female farmers who are looking out for the interests of small farmers, gardeners, and health-conscious people.

Here is a direct quote from CommonGround's website:

"Consumers aren't getting the real story about American agriculture and all that goes into growing and raising their food. We're a group of volunteer farm women and we plan to change that by doing something extraordinary. Our program is called CommonGround and it's all about starting a conversation between women who grow food, and the women who buy it. It's a conversation based on our personal experience as farmers, but also on science and research. Our first goal is to help consumers understand that their food is not grown by a factory. It's grown by people and it's important to us that you understand and trust the process. We hope you'll join in the conversation." [57]

This is another truly impressive site, downplaying virtually any harm to humans or the environment that results from Industrial Ag practices.

But who is the creator of CommonGround's message?

When I originally wrote this section last year, CommonGround's website was registered on www.WhoIs.com to Jack Lawry at Osborn & Barr Communications in St. Louis, Missouri.[56]

O & B specializes in conventional agricultural marketing and PR, which includes the creation of front groups for their clients. The United Soybean Board happens to be one of O & B's clients, as well as Merk Animal Health, and Monsanto—their largest.[58,59]

Interestingly, Monsanto hired O & B in 2006 to help quell consumer concerns regarding the Recombinant Bovine Growth Hormone (rBGH used in cattle) issue. Toward that end, O & B created a pro-rBGH farmer front group called *American Farmers for Advancement and Conservation of Technology* (AFACT: www.itisafact.org).[60,61]

So whether CommonGround's message sponsors are limited to The United Soybean Board and The National Corn Growers Association, it's hard to say, but my guess is that Monsanto is also part of this front group.

NOTE: www.whois.com now says www.findourcommonground.com registrant is "registration private," protected by domainsbyproxy.com.[62] But since I referenced the O & B connection myself, I know it's accurate. AND I learned a lesson—now I take a screen shot if I think the sponsors may remove implicating information.

And Two More, Grander-Scale Examples of Front Groups:

Rick Berman, Lawyer, Lobbyist, and King of Front Groups: AKA "Dr. Evil"

No joke, that's what people call him.

With Corporate money paying for Berman's services (Berman & Co., www.bermanco.com), he wages war on consumer safety groups, environmental advocate groups, animal rights groups, unions. You name it. Rick Berman's entire goal is to create doubt in your mind, at least, and find an ally in you, at best.

This man leads more than 40 Industry-sponsored front groups and projects therein. He's a one-man wrecking machine! There is an entire website dedicated to revealing his deceptive endeavors. Check it out at: www.bermanexposed.org.

One major Dr. Evil-created front group that revolves around food and water issues is *The Center for Consumer Freedom,* which is, of course, sponsored by the food and beverage Industry.[63] This front group has many projects at work including: three websites downplaying the dangers of mercury in fish, three propagating misinformation regarding animal cruelty, one spewing propaganda regarding health care research, and another disregarding the evidence linking obesity to high fructose corn syrup. Oh, and there is another website that is devoted exclusively to disparaging the *Center* for *Science in the Public Interest* (CSPI), a health and nutrition organization.

The *Center for Consumer Freedom* website states they are "A nonprofit organization devoted to promoting personal responsibility and protecting consumer choices. We believe that the consumer is King. And Queen." They claim that a growing number of health advocates and environmental activists now "meddle in Americans' lives... They all claim to know 'what's best for you'... In reality, they're eroding our basic freedoms..."[64] Yee Gods!

If you'd like to watch his story, there is a great video by MSNBC called *Meet Rick Berman*, which you can find on You Tube or www.lighten yourtoxicload.com.

And last (for now), but certainly not least:

<u>Citizens United</u>

Citizens United is perhaps *The Mother* of all front groups. It's a very misleading name for a non-profit organization funded by a conservative group of right-wing-bagillionaires whose true intention is to promote corporate profit *and* the candidates who endorse their agendas.

Because they have greatly benefited from Citizens United's efforts, this organization has been connected to the Koch Brothers.[65,66] The Koch Brothers are the owners of Koch Industries (with hands in everything from oil refineries to Brawny® paper towels), which was named the second largest private company by *Forbes* in 2013.[2] The Koch Brothers are linked to funding Tea Party groups, as well as *Americans for Prosperity*, *FreedomWorks*, and *Citizens for a Sound Economy.*[67]

The Koch Brothers—tying Bill Gates for the #1 richest person in America at a net worth of $72 *billion*[68]—are big proponents of less government regulation (specifically with regard to their Industries and activities) and more Corporate control (of things like public information and our right to free speech).[69]

Citizens United shares the same goals as the Koch Brothers, of course, although you wouldn't quite gather that from their carefully chosen name or the description found on the website. To gather a more accurate picture of the actual agenda, I found it helps to replace the word "citizen" with "Corporate/Corporations":

"**Citizens** United is an organization dedicated to restoring our government to **citizens'** control. Through a combination of education, advocacy, and grass roots organization, **Citizens** United seeks to reassert the traditional American values of limited government, freedom of enterprise, strong families, and national sovereignty and security. **Citizens** United's goal is to restore the founding father's vision of a free nation, guided by the honesty, common sense, and good will of its **citizens.**"[70]

In a 2010 Supreme Court case *Citizens United vs. Federal Election*

Commission (which determines election rules and campaign funding laws), the judges ruled in favor of Citizens United. In a nutshell, this ruling determined that Corporations have a Constitutional right to freedom of speech (essentially giving Corporations the same rights as an individual citizen, otherwise known as "corporate personhood"), while also granting Corporations free reign for unlimited spending to influence elections in order to promote the candidates who will support their agendas. This decision not only overruled the standing Federal Election Commission policies, but also successfully overturned more-than-a-century-old precedent that was signed into law by President Theodore Roosevelt, which prohibited Corporations from making any campaign contributions *whatsoever*, for any direct *or indirect* political purpose. You know, for the exact purpose of ensuring that Corporations were not buying politicians. Not that it helped to the degree intended, but at least there was some sort of standard in place.

Unfortunately, this Citizens United, most likely Koch-sponsored victory, was just one more step toward shutting an unwitting public out of its own government. So beware of this group, their deceptive name, and the people involved, because unless you are part of the wealthiest 1%, they are most definitely not looking out for YOU.

However, thankfully, some of our politicians are:

"Our elections no longer focus on the best ideas, but the biggest bank accounts, and Americans' right to free speech should not be determined by their net worth. I am proud to be introducing this amendment [Campaign Finance Reform] to change the way we do business in Washington and get money out of a broken system that puts special interest over people."[71]
—*SENATOR TOM UDALL (D-N.M.)*

THE BOTTOM LINE

Same-same. Be sure to watch for message sponsors—and unless you trust and *know* your source—take everything you read, hear, or watch with 10,000 grains of salt! You've got to ask yourself: Who is the *true* source of this information, and what is their motivation? If you don't know, don't believe 'em.

TO LEARN MORE ABOUT FRONT GROUPS, TRANSPARENCY IN FUNDING, AND FOLLOWING THE PAPER TRAIL, YOU CAN VISIT:

- www.sourcewatch.org/index.php/Portal:Front_groups
- www.followthemoney.org/
- www.sourcewatch.org/index.php/SourceWatch:How_to_research_front_groups

And by the way, Pro-Industry sources claim that these types of reference sites, ones intending to create transparency, are sites run by extremist way-too-far-to-the-left liberals. Yes, there is definitely a democratic filter. And while the extreme-liberal-accusation may even be true, that does not mean the information isn't accurate or useful. Please know, however, that some of these sites do rely on public content that, although cited, you would be wise to fact-check on your own. These sites are somewhat *of the people, by the people, for the people.* But that certainly does not mean that the content is propaganda or urban myth. How else will we ever uncover the facts if we don't work together?

Opposed-to-these-sites folks also point to the funding sources for organizations such as *SourceWatch,* which is run by *The Center for Media and Democracy.* Yes, many of these sites are sustained by grant money and donations, which often comes from people, trusts, or foundations who obviously share the same motivations for transparency, democratic freedom, and helping humanity. And yes, this money provides operating capital and money to pay staff. But what business, organization, or service doesn't require money to run? Every organization that I count on and trust to provide truthful information relies on outside funding.

In my experience, the motivations behind these perhaps way-too-far-to-the-left liberal sites and organizations are noble and in service to creating a greater life for all, not just the few. This is in direct opposition, of course, to self-serving motivations based on profit and greed.

The reality is: Everyone has an agenda, but not all are equal.

Please know that Big Biz and their proponents will do everything they can to convince you that activists and people attempting to help preserve our democratic rights are quacks, conspiracy theorists, fanatics, and even national security threats (when what they really mean is *Corporate* security threat). Folks will say anything to protect their empires— or hire "reputable" sources to say anything—to convince you they are right.

I am simply sharing information. I'll leave it up to you to decide what to believe and whom to trust.

Aside from Corporations funding their own safety studies and throwing all kinds of BIG money at the propagation of Pro-Industry information, there is another Burly-Brazen-Beast used by Corporations to bulldoze their agendas along—a highly dysfunctional species known as *Lobbyists*.

LOBBYING

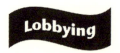

The laws, legislations, and government favors that help keep Big Biz running the show are won and held in place with the help of Corporate Lobbyists. Lobbyists play a very key role in keeping Big Pharma, Chem, Ag, and Food in command, and they are *extremely* good at their jobs. And there's also a whole lot of them hanging around Washington! In fact, according to *The Center for Responsive Politics*, there were an estimated 12,278 lobbyists working their magic on the system in 2013![72]

Lobbying is the stage where our government really begins to join the Corporate-greed game.

What Exactly is a Lobbyist?

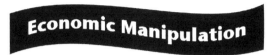

Typically, a lobbyist is a highly-paid person whose job is to convince Congress, lawmakers, and the heads of our Public Agencies to pass legislation in favor of their client's interests. Often, their clients are the BIG Corporations/Industries.

Although unethical *and illegal*, many lobbyists bribe politicians and lawmakers with money, job offers, extravagant gifts, special treatment—whatever gets the job done—in order to swing rules and regulations in support of their Corporate client's agenda.

It is very important to note, however, that not all lobbyists are unethical or highly paid. Some lobbyists are volunteers that work for independent non-profit, grassroots organizations that are truly working for the good of the whole. But, of course, these do-gooder folks are not the ones with whom we are concerned.

Jack Abramoff, on the other hand—holy moly! Straight from the horse's mouth, his story will tell you everything you need to know about the corrupt world of Corporate Lobbyists.

Jack Abramoff: An Infamous Lobbyist
Spills the Beans

In the 1990s, Jack Abramoff mastered the art of showering gifts on lawmakers in exchange for their votes on legislation and tax breaks for his clients. His influence in government was so pervasive that he alone controlled about a quarter of the U.S. Congress! In fact, Abramoff was so proficient at his job that he took home $20 million a year.

After serving 3½ years in prison (not for bribing Congressmen mind you, but for tax evasion and ripping off his own clients), Abramoff came forward to reveal the disturbing truth about what can (and does) take place between Corporate Lobbyists and Lawmakers.

This is an unbelievable account produced by *60 Minutes*. If you haven't seen it, *please* watch it! You can find it on You Tube or www.lightenyourtoxicload.com: *Jack Abramoff—The Lobbyist's Playbook*. This video explains the reality of lobbying far better than my words ever could.

HOW MUCH MONEY IS SPENT ON LOBBYING FOR FAVORABLE LEGISLATION AND TAX BREAKS?

Two examples of *reported* spending on lobbying:

- In 2013, the Pharmaceutical/Health Products Industry dispensed nearly $226 million, making it the largest Industry lobby in the U.S. at this time.[73] Pharmaceutical Research & Manufacturers of America was the largest contributor, spending almost $18 million of the lobbying total, followed by Eli Lily & Co, Amgen, and Pfizer.[74]

- In 2013, Big Ag forked over $149.5+ million, making it the 8th most powerful economic sector and growing since 2010.[75] "Food processing & Sales" was the largest contributor to the overall lobby total, spending over $39.6 million. Grocery Manufacturers Association (GMA), Nestle, General Mills, and Kraft are the four largest clients within the "Food processing & Sales" lobby,[76] all very large proponents of junk foods and GMOs.

  "Agricultural Services/Products" is the second largest contributor to the Big Ag lobby, spending $35.8 million. Monsanto, American Farm Bureau, and Crop Life America are the three largest clients in this segment,[77] all in favor of GMOs, pesticides, and the like.

Check it out! **www.opensecrets.org/lobby/index.php**

"The primary goal of much of the money that flows through U.S. politics is this: Influence. Corporations and industry groups, labor unions, single-issue organizations—together, they spend billions of dollars each year to gain access to decision-makers in government, all in an attempt to influence their thinking."
—*OPEN SECRETS.ORG, CENTER FOR RESPONSIVE POLITICS*[78]

THE "REVOLVING DOOR"

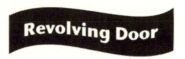

Okay, so let's do a small recap.

In order to accomplish their money-grubbing goals, Corporations sponsor their own research, financially motivate those willing to sell out in the "scientific" community, hire lobbyists to keep their selfish interests in charge, and use PR firms and front groups to manipulate and confuse consumers. In addition, we have another very commonly practiced phenomenon called the "revolving door." Now, we've got all the BIG players in bed with one another, giving each other massages, scratching each other's backs, and sharing cigarettes made of gold.

What is the Revolving Door?

In politics, the "revolving door" is defined as: The shuffling of personnel between public positions in government and private positions in Industry. A person may actually spend his/her entire career in revolving door activity, spinning in and out of private and public sectors.

To understand what this actually means and why it matters, let's take a closer look at the mechanics. The process can work a couple of different ways:

An individual starts out in a government position—a Congressman or the head of the FDA, for example. Then, Industry hires that government official for a Corporate career—V.P. of Sales for a pharmaceutical company, for instance—when his/her term is completed.

But here's the kicker:

Government officials are often secured for future Industry careers while _still in office_.

No potential conflict of interest here, right? Riiiiiiiggghhhttt.

This pre-meditated arrangement means that in exchange for high-paying employment offers—which often double to triple their salaries—Industry has the ability to develop relationships with government officials in order to secure favorable legislation, regulation, and government contracts. Furthermore, these incestuous relationships give Industry an opportunity to gather inside intel on government happenings.

According to a featured article in _Republic Report_:

"Our research effort uncovered the partial salaries of 12 lawmakers-turned-lobbyists. Republic Report's _investigation found that lawmakers increased their salary by 1,452 percent on average from the last year they were in office to the latest publicly available disclosure."_[79]

71

The revolving door can also work in reverse:

An individual starts out in an Industry position—maybe a lobbyist, consultant, or strategist. Then, government appoints that Industry professional for a government post—such as a Senior Policy Advisor to a Senator or a U.S. Representative.

Government usually hires from Industry to capitalize on Corporate influence, power, and money. This is especially true when government endeavors to do business with or regulate a Corporation. But government may also hire from Industry in order to secure political support—in the form of campaign contributions, donations, or endorsements—from private firms.

Industry professionals benefit from government hire by moving into a position that, once again, can make it very easy to pass laws that favor the Corporation in which they either: have a vested interest, are still working for, or will return to when their term in office is completed. In any of these scenarios, these individuals often reap huge financial rewards from pulling strings while in office that support their Industry's success.

Government wins. Industry wins.
Everybody involved profits from the revolving relationship.
Except you and me, of course.

The Revolving Door in Motion

As we will see in following chapters, the revolving door is pervasive in our political system. For now, as a living example of the revolving door in motion, we'll look at the bio of a lady named Linda Fisher.[80] I honestly have never heard of her, and I am guessing you probably haven't either. That is precisely why I chose her. Being a neutral example, there are no preconceived notions about her motivations. It's just the facts.

Here's Fisher's career history:

- **Public Sector**: For 10 years, Linda Fisher worked for the U.S. Environmental Protection Agency (EPA), holding a handful of different positions but most notably, "Assistant Administrator — Office of Prevention, Pesticides, and Toxic Substances."

  - ✓ **And Private**: From 1993 to 1995, while working for the EPA, Fisher was also "Of Counsel" with the law firm *Latham & Watkins*, which represents "public and private life science companies," including those within the Biotechnology and Pharmaceutical Industries.[81]

- **Private**: Subsequently, from 1995 to 2000, Fisher served as the Vice President of Government Affairs for Monsanto Company, the infamous pesticide and biotechnology Corporation we keep hearing so much about.

  - ✓ Fisher was also a member of a USDA advisory committee on biotech foods.[82]

- **Public**: In 2001 to 2003, Fisher went back to a government position at the EPA as Deputy Administrator.

- **Private**: In 2004 she went to work for DuPont as the "Vice President, Safety, Health & Environment Chief Sustainability Officer," which is a position listed on the site under "DuPont and the Government."[83]

DuPont, remember, is one of the Big Six Chemical manufacturers, and the agriculture division of DuPont makes and sells genetically modified seeds for GMO crops.

So, the question is, is Linda Fisher and her revolving door activity proof of a conflict of interest? We don't know for sure. Has she been pulling strings in her government positions to support employers such as Monsanto and DuPont? Maybe, but it's hard to say. Is she interested in protecting the environment or the Biotech and Chemical Industries? Good question.

If you Google Fisher, she appears to be geared toward environmental care and sustainability. However, her employment history, jumping back and forth between the Environmental Protection Agency, Monsanto, and DuPont—major Biotech Corporations and direct manufacturers of poisons that are toxic to our soil, water, animals, and us—sure begs the question, where do her loyalties *actually* lie? And that, my friend, is the very big issue with revolving door activity.

In this dizzying and complicated revolving door phenomenon, sussing out who's who, where they came from, where they are going, and whose team they're on, is a confusing and sticky web, just as it is intended to be.

A Word about Congress, Lobbyists, and the Revolving Door

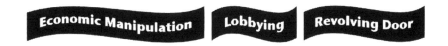

In case you haven't guessed, lobbying, the revolving door, and Congress are three peas in a pod. Because when it comes to influencing policy and regulations, the main asset for a lobbyist is contact with and influence over government officials. Through lobbying and revolving door activity, Corporations can assure that influential individuals are in the perfect policy-making position in government, at the exact right time, to achieve their goals.

How do they get away with these shenanigans?

Money, Power, and Secrecy.

These deals between Congress and Corporate lobbyists are obviously not public information. For example, legislators can pass laws or generate special tax breaks that benefit their future employer with very-little-to-zero accountability or transparency.

So how can we raise a stink if we don't even know this stuff is happening? Well, that's all changing now, isn't it?

You can look up any member of Congress, lobbying, and revolving door activity here: www.opensecrets.org/revolving/index.php.

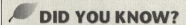

DID YOU KNOW?

OpenSecrets database lists 421 former members of Congress involved in revolving door activity.[84]

THE BOTTOM LINE

Due to major conflicts of interest and lack of transparency, the revolving door between Industry and government can—and does—lead to promoting Corporate Interests over public health and freedom.

Two More Final Corporate-Agenda-Making Tactics

When the tried-and-true-tactics are not quite enough to accomplish their agenda, or they need to slow a process down, Corporations have a couple of other tricks in their bag.

Sometimes they'll use:

DELAY TACTICS

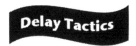

When Corporations need to buy time, delay tactics are the go-to option.

To instigate delay, a Corporation might initiate a lawsuit, fund parallel studies, swamp researchers in administrative procedures, demand different peer reviews, or instigate congressional inquiries.

Delay tactics can be exceptionally fruitful when trying to slow or suppress the release of unfavorable study results, influence scientific evidence, or gain commercial advantage. Delay tactics can also be used to manipulate political procedures—when a statute of limitations is involved in an impending investigation for example, or during election time when incoming administrations (perhaps Corporation-planted via lobbying or the revolving door) will undoubtedly support the Corporate goals that hang in the balance.

"Studies of life-science faculty indicate that researchers with industry funding are more likely to withhold research results in order to secure commercial advantage."[85]
—*INTEGRITY IN SCIENCE PROJECT, CSPI*

We will see some great examples of well-timed delay tactics used by the Food Industry in the next chapter.

And last, but certainly not least, there is always…

HARASSMENT

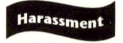

Parties with a vested interest in success have been known to harass, silence, or fire an individual attempting to publicize undesirable information or unfavorable study results. These amazingly courageous people are often referred to as "whistleblowers."

If an individual cannot legally be fired for whatever reason, sometimes that person is humiliated or shunned so severely, he/she resigns. Unfortunately, this tactic appears to be relatively common right now in our highly dysfunctional food system.

One example is Dr. Arpad Pusztai, a Hungarian-born biochemist, nutritionist, and Fellow of the Royal Society of Edinburgh. After conducting a study on genetically modified potatoes, Dr. Pusztai revealed that his results showed dangerous implications for human health. As a consequence, he was forced to retire from his position of 35 years at the *Rowett Institute of Nutrition and Health.* He tells his story in *Scientists Under Attack,* which can be found at: www.scientistsunderattack.com

"To learn who rules over you, simply find out who you are not allowed to criticize."
—VOLTAIRE

BUT WHAT ABOUT THE FDA?
ISN'T IT THEIR JOB TO PROTECT US?

You bet your sweet bippy! Protecting the public is the very reason for their existence. Just for fun, let's take a peek at the FDA's Mission Statement:

"The FDA is responsible for protecting the public health by assuring the safety, efficacy, and security of human and veterinary drugs, biological products, medical devices, our nation's food supply, cosmetics, and products that emit radiation. The FDA is also responsible for advancing the public health by helping to speed innovations that make medicines and foods more effective, safer, and more affordable; and helping the public get the accurate, science-based information they need to use medicines and foods to improve their health."[86]

After reading that statement, all I can say is: Wow, they sure seem to be falling short of their mark.

But as I have mentioned along the way, the FDA—being a government agency—is highly vulnerable to all of the Corporate Machinations discussed in this chapter. And, of course, this can have huge implications for the hasty approval of products-not-yet-proven-safe, as well as the tortoise-like manner in which harmful substances are removed from the marketplace.

The FDA and Big Pharma

It is important to note that ties between the FDA and the Pharmaceutical Industry are particularly strong. So much so that Big Pharma—and thus Big Chem—is funding an outrageously large percentage of the FDA's annual budget.

In fact, according to the FDA, and this is probably a conservative estimate, Big Pharma companies now provide 60% of the FDA's drug review costs via "user fees." How much funding are we talking about here? Well, something around the tune of a whopping *$718.7 million* per year, the exact amount that the FDA projected they would rake in from drug company "user fees" in 2013!![87]

That's a helluva lotta cake! And slightly disturbing. But let's back up for a second, because you might be wondering…

What Are "User Fees?"

User fees are monies paid to the FDA, by a drug company, for the review and approval of a new pharmaceutical drug.

But not just any ol' drug. The drug company is paying the FDA to review and approve a drug that *they* created and plan to sell. As quickly as possible, I might add.

A Pharma-funded FDA sounds like a terrible idea to me, especially at first blush, but there are definitely potential pros *and* cons, which are important to note.

On the sunnier side, as the pro-argument goes, user fees provide the funding to expedite the review and approval of pharmaceuticals, which becomes extremely important when a drug could potentially cure a rare disease. Also, the extra funding may actually, as claimed, help support a more thorough review process, which may keep drugs-that-eventually-prove-dangerous off the market in the first place. Both of these points are huge potential positives.

On the cloudier-con-side of the argument, however, an expedited approval process could also mean just the opposite—dangerous, not-thoroughly-tested drugs may simply be approved more quickly. Which leads us to the real issue here: There is a rather large and looming potential for conflicts of interest. If Big Pharma is paying the FDA's bills, where will the FDA's loyalty lie when the rubber hits the road?

And No, This Is Not the Way the System Used to Work...

Until 1992, the U.S. Treasury provided funding for the review and regulation of prescription drugs. No Private Industry was involved. The funding model simply used government (taxpayer) money to fund a government agency process.

Then, as a response to Big Pharma's complaints that the drug review and approval process took too long—that their drugs were not approved quickly enough—PDUFA (Prescription Drug User Fee Act) was passed. And poof! The FDA's review and approval of pharmaceutical drugs is now (and has been for the last 11+ years) largely sponsored by the Pharmaceutical Companies themselves.

So now, Big Pharma Companies—those with a highly vested interest in the approval and subsequent sale of their product—are not only conducting their own research studies, they are also providing direct cash funding to the FDA to "Ensure Drugs Are Safe and Effective," too.

And now I think to myself—again—Big Pharma involved in the regulatory process? Seriously??! Even considering the *potential* positives, does that really seem like a good idea?

And it's important to remember, user fees probably aren't the only source of money flowing through the FDA from Big Pharma, although the most transparent for sure. Big Pharma also has a *monstrous* lobby that can feed a luxury-hungry FDA official a smorgasbord of other lucrative—and much more difficult to track—sources of bonus income.

And don't forget the ubiquitous revolving door! High-ranking FDA officials can secure extremely profitable consulting positions within the Pharmaceutical Industry they were previously regulating when they leave the FDA, or vice-versa. *Open Secrets: Center for Responsive Politics* lists 65 people revolving between Big Pharma and the FDA.[88] Of course, not every individual listed has engaged in shady activity, but the work histories of many folks sure do scream "conflict of interest!"

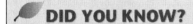 **DID YOU KNOW?**

As of 2009, the global market for pharmaceuticals was worth over $837 billion, and is projected to reach over $1 *trillion* in 2014.[89]

"Perhaps 'FDA' really stands for Fatal Drugs Allowed?"
—DR. BETTY MARTINI, ASPARTAME ACTIVIST[90]

Unfortunately, pharmaceutical drugs are promoted as the answer to all of our health problems. Often dodgy drugs, I might add.

How 'bout those television commercials selling you a fluffy fantasy of health, happiness, and sex appeal while simultaneously reciting a rapid-fire, monotonic, almost-cheerful-chant that supposedly intends to warn you of the horrific litany of potential side-effects? Death, suicide, bleeding ulcers, heart attack, stroke? *Really*??! Those commercials make me wonder if the mainstream American public is so thoroughly brainwashed that they think those things will never happen or couldn't possibly be true?

Oh, but they are true. And they do happen. Sometimes the FDA approves very dangerous—even deadly—drugs. What's more, as the years go by, adverse effects and deaths seem to increase:

- In 2006, Dr. David Graham—*Associate Director of the FDA's Office of Drug Safety*—while speaking about the drug *Vioxx* (pulled from the market in 2004), the FDA, and ties to Big Pharma, reports:

  "The FDA is responsible for 140,000 heart attacks and 60,000 dead Americans. That's as many people as were killed in the Vietnam War. Yet the FDA points the finger at me and says, 'Well, this guy's a rat, you can't trust him,' but nobody is calling them to account. Congress isn't calling them to account. For the American people, it's dropped off the radar screen. They should be screaming because this can happen again." [91]

- In 2007, according to reports by the FDA, the Centers for Disease Control and Prevention (CDC), and the U.S. Consumer Product Safety Commission, more than 700,000 Americans end up in emergency rooms each year due to harmful reactions to even some of the most commonly prescribed medicines—such as insulin and antibiotics.[92]

- In 2008, almost 50,000 Americans died, and there were 320,000 serious adverse effects reported to the FDA due to pharmaceutical drugs.[93,94]

  NOTE: The FDA estimates that less than 1% of all serious adverse events are actually reported directly to the agency.[95]

- In 2011, an analysis by the *Institute of Safe Medicine Practices* (ISMP) estimated 2 to 4 million persons suffered serious, disabling, or fatal reactions associated with prescription drugs— including 128,000 patient deaths—based on a full year of reports to the FDA.[95]

DOCUMENTARY: If you'd like to get an inside scoop on the Pharmaceutical Industry and the FDA, Dr. Gary Null's *Prescription for Disaster* video is a go-to source. You can find it on Amazon.[96]

DID YOU KNOW?

According to a report from Public Citizen, "The pharmaceutical industry now tops not only the defense industry, but all other industries in the total amount of fraud payments for actions against the federal government under the False Claims Act."[97]

The two main violations? Illegal off-label promotion of pharmaceuticals and deliberately overcharging state health programs (mainly Medicaid).

It may come as no surprise, but the large Big Pharma Corporations rarely face criminal charges, regardless of fraud, death caused by unsafe drugs, off-label promotion (promoting a drug for un-approved use), or other unlawful activity. They may get sued or pay a chunky fine, but what is that but a slap on the wrist when fines are most likely a key element of their financial planning?

This is a tangled web complicated by Medicare and Medicaid, whose laws, in a nutshell, forbid them to do business with fraudulent, criminal companies.[98,99] As it should be, right? Yes, of course, in an ideal world. However, in our drug-dependent culture, Medicare and Medicaid apparently can't live without Big Pharma. So at least for now, criminal prosecution is not really an option.

It seems that Big Pharma has also been successfully skirting prosecution by misusing the 1st Amendment, claiming free speech in their illegal off-label promotions.[100,101]

The FDA Itself States the Need for Agency Reform

The U.S. government is, of course, well aware of these issues, as stated in their own 2007 report "FDA Science and Mission at Risk."[102]

Simply taking a peek at the table of contents of this 60-page report tells a big chunk of the story.

For instance, "Major Findings" include:

- "The FDA cannot fulfill its mission because its scientific base has eroded and its scientific organizational structure is weak."

- "The FDA cannot fulfill its mission because its scientific workforce does not have sufficient capacity and capability."

And in the "Discussion of Key Findings and Recommendations" section you'll find statements such as:

- "FDA does not have the capacity to ensure the safety of food for the nation."

- "The development of medical products based on 'new science' cannot adequately be regulated by the FDA."

- "The FDA lacks the information science capability and information infrastructure to fulfill its regulatory mandate."

Enough said? I think so. I can virtually guarantee very little has changed since 2007. After all, another nickname for the FDA is *Foot Dragging Artists*. And you will see how true this nickname is as our adventure unfolds.

The FDA, Big Pharma, and Natural Supplements

Of utmost importance to note, the FDA, with all of its substandard safety and slippery regulatory policies of pharmaceutical drugs, regularly attacks the alternative health care industry. Pretty much anything natural that doesn't feed Big Pharma or Big Chem—like organic foods, nutritional supplements, herbs, minerals, or alternative healing modalities that support our bodies' natural propensity for optimal health—is vigorously criticized, reported as dangerous, or considered quackery.

The FDA, along with Corporate-Sponsored Information, has successfully manufactured a culture of fear and doubt with regard to nutritional supplements and alternative health options—while pushing the public to blindly swallow sometimes dangerous, albeit "approved" drugs. This is not a mystery: The FDA is clearly biased in favor of pharmaceutical drugs over natural alternatives.

As such, the Big-Pharma-fueled-FDA has been trying to pull nutritional supplements and herbs off the shelves for years. Since they have yet to succeed, Big Pharma is now attempting to sneak in through the back door and take control of natural options by purchasing nutritional supplement companies. For example, Bayer Health Care LLC was slated to purchase Schiff Nutrition International, a large nutritional supplement company, by the end of 2012.[103] Thank God, Buddha, Allah, Jehovah... to whomever you pray... the deal fell through because supplement takeover by Big Pharma could be very bad news. Here's why.

If Big Pharma gains control of the natural supplement industry, new legislation will likely treat vitamins, minerals, and herbs as "medical drugs." This means that availability, affordability, and dosage efficacy would be subject to "government" regulation. In other words, if Big Pharma takes over the natural supplement industry, you may lose your ability to pop over to your local health food store to pick up your favorite cold remedy or arthritis supplement, because you may be required to have a prescription. Or the dosage will be so low it may be ineffective, or the price will be so high, you may not be able to afford them—or all of the above.

As we discussed, pharmaceuticals don't have the best track record. While on the flip side, natural remedies have been used and proven safe for centuries, with very few adverse or harmful reactions. In fact, according to a "U.S. National Poison Data System" 2010 annual report, data from 57 U.S. poison centers showed that out of 1,366 reported deaths, a total of *zero* deaths were caused by vitamin and mineral supplements, while pharmaceutical drugs caused more than 1,100 deaths![104]

THE BOTTOM LINE

Big Pharma doesn't want you to have free access to natural supplements or alternative health care because these options are highly effective and Big Pharma doesn't currently control them. They would much rather feed you pharmaceuticals than have you find ways to be well on our own, because if you are well, they don't make money.

Life-supporting foods, clean water, herbs, supplements, and alternative health care are incredibly powerful tools that promote health and healing for the body, mind, and spirit.

CAN SUPPLEMENTS BE HARMFUL?

The quality of natural supplements is incredibly important. Not all supplements are created equally. And not all are beneficial for everyone. Furthermore, supplements that are considered hazardous usually—often illegally—contain some type of pharmaceutical or synthetic ingredient. With that said, exercising caution with the high-energy, fat-burning, diet, and muscle-building variety of products, is probably wise.

It's always best to consult a reputable alternative health care provider to help you design a lifestyle plan that is tailored to your individual needs and goals. Each one of us has our own unique requirements when it comes to diet, exercise, or health-supporting supplements.

You can visit www.lightenyourtoxicload.com to see some of my favorite products and trusted brands, as well as a growing directory of alternative healthcare practitioners to help guide you on your path to optimal health.

IN CLOSING

Remember to always keep in mind: Through ginormous amounts of money and power, our right to straightforward, honest information—and true democracy—is hijacked when Corporate Greed is running the show. And Corporate Greed IS currently running the show—and our government.

However…

IT'S TIME TO TAKE THE POWER BACK!

While the political situation may seem dire, we are not helpless. In the past, you may have succumbed to the idea that there is nothing you can do about the state of your health, our nation, and the planet, but I am here to tell you that those limiting, lazy-making beliefs are simply not true!

However, the solution IS up to you. And me. And each one of our neighbors. Taking responsibility *and* action is absolutely necessary to create positive change.

A Positive and Proactive Perspective

It's important to note that the political landscape, at least to some degree, is really trying to evolve for the better. There have always been very caring people in office, and running for office, who truly want to help return to a more functional, fair, sustainable system that cares for people over profit. These individuals are The Champions within our system—bless their courageous hearts—who definitely need our support *and* our votes. As we move along, you will be learning more about lawmakers and regulators who stand for YOU, not Big Business.

But we can't really *wait* for the system to change. Because as we've learned in this chapter, as the system stands right now, we, unfortunately, cannot count on the government as a whole to look out for our health, well-being, and freedom. Furthermore, solutions to bring about substantial and lasting change will (most likely) not be found in reform efforts, because the majority of the very people in charge of creating—and enforcing—reform policies are also the ones who greatly benefit from things staying exactly as they are. Borrowing from a quote by Upton Sinclair: "It is difficult to get a person to enforce something when his/her income depends upon not enforcing it."

THE REALLY GOOD NEWS!

First, the politics of food are obviously driven by Money. Money, money, money. That means you and I—the Consumers—are actually the ones in control. If we don't buy, they don't sell. If they don't sell, they don't make money. That means that each and every day, you drive the market—and the political platform—**by what you choose to buy and buy *into***. Pretty simple, really!

Second, regardless of the goals of Corporate-Greedheads and Fat-Cat groups like Citizens United, we still live in a democracy. However, your right to receive unbiased information, and therefore your freedom to make healthy choices, is obviously at stake, so keeping your eyes and ears open is vitally important. NOW is the time to dust off any apathy that you may have collected over the years, and choose to become savvy, awake, aware, and vocal. If you are willing to pay a little bit of attention, you can help stop sneaky legislations and tactics before they slip through cracks.

Do not underestimate the power of your pocketbook or your voice. Both are invaluable ways to change policy. Rest assured, in numbers, we *can* create a healthier, happier system for all.

"Democracy belongs to those who exercise it."
—BILL MOYERS

THE GOAL

To reach a "tipping point": When a critical mass of citizens refuse unnecessary and often dangerous drugs and toxic food and demand that our public servants stop serving Corporate Interests over public health and well-being.

WHAT YOU CAN DO RIGHT NOW

- If you haven't done so already, please watch the Jack Abramoff video about Corporate Lobbyists. This is a very important concept to understand.

- Keep reading! Education creates awareness, which illuminates choices and promotes action.

- Sign up for email alerts and breaking news reports from independent sources that are hard at work to help keep you up to speed with the latest information on important issues.

- ✓ You can find abundant links to my most trusted resources at www.lightenyourtoxicload.com under "Take Action."

- ✓ You can also follow my blog for important updates and action alerts.

- Sign and forward public petitions that arrive via email alerts. Signing petitions is the **easiest way to use your voice. It's free and only takes a few seconds**. Petitions are a fantastic tool to help create change. Remember, the power is in the numbers, so don't think for a single second that your signature doesn't matter. If a petition issue speaks to you, just sign it!

- If you have the means, please help support these independent organizations that tirelessly fight for your rights and keep you informed. They are kept alive through donations, and they really need our financial aid to continue doing their amazing work.

NEXT CHAPTER

We'll take a look at the approval history of the artificial sweetener, *aspartame*. As the most contentious food additive ever created, aspartame is the perfect case study of *The Politics of Food*. Get ready to be shocked! This is stranger than fiction.

"For what is a man profited, if he shall gain the whole world, and lose his own soul?"
—MATHEW 16:26

CHAPTER 3:

Aspartame

A CASE STUDY ON THE POLITICS OF FOOD

"The problem with aspartame, includes not only the biochemical nature of this toxin, but also sheds light on the political nature of the players involved and the changes in regulatory policies and regulations resulting from corporate-government ties and the politicians closely associated with these ties."
—*ARTHUR M. EVANGELISTA, DIRECTOR OF OPERATIONS, FORMER FDA INVESTIGATOR*

A WORD OF ENCOURAGEMENT

The approval of the artificial sweetener "aspartame"—and its continued use in multitudes of "sugar-free" and "diet" products today—is a perfect example of *The Politics of Food* at work. This is a long but very important, real-life drama, so please try to stick with me until the very end! And remember to consume this information slowly, in bite-sized pieces, so as to give yourself time to digest the density.

Believe it or not, entire books have been written on the subject of aspartame. And during my research on this subject, I have encountered my fair share of confusing information. With that said, I have done my absolute best to accurately dissect the essential details of this information-dense topic to create a relatively easy read. Consequently, I have not covered every facet, issue, or argument with regard to aspartame's history or health concerns. I'm guessing that most people would rather have the *Reader's Digest* version, in this fast-paced, I'd-rather-watch-a-90-second-YouTube-video culture in which we now reside.

We will conclude this chapter with some basic information about what aspartame is actually made of, the various health issues associated with its consumption, and how to avoid it.

STRANGER THAN FICTION

The aspartame story is truly the stuff of movies. Had I not done the research myself, I would've never believed this shameful drama could actually be true. I was pleased to discover that most of the hard facts in this case are substantiated in Congressional Records and Senate Hearings, much of which you can find at www.lightenyourtoxicload.com, along with other supporting material.

As the details of this account unfolded, I was (once again) repeatedly astonished to learn the depth of deceit that can happen behind closed doors—secret skeletons held hostage, hidden from public awareness. Until brave individuals pry the door open, that is, and set the spirits of transparency free.

NOTHING SHORT OF CRIMINAL

Economic Manipulation

Aspartame's lengthy history is tainted, every step of the way, by decisions that were (and still are) strictly financially and politically motivated and completely under Corporate Control.

Using many of the tactics you learned in Chapter Two, G.D. Searle Co. (pharmaceutical company and the makers of aspartame) successfully manipulated, bribed, and infiltrated government agencies, congress, research institutions, and organizations that we have all been taught to trust. We will see a firsthand example of how unchecked Corporate Power can successfully conceal criminal activity, lies, and fraud.

As *60 Minutes* correspondent Mike Wallace stated in a 1996 interview: The approval of aspartame was "the most contested in FDA history."[1] Why? Because the approval process was nothing short of scandalous.

THE MIND-BOGGLING
HISTORY OF ASPARTAME

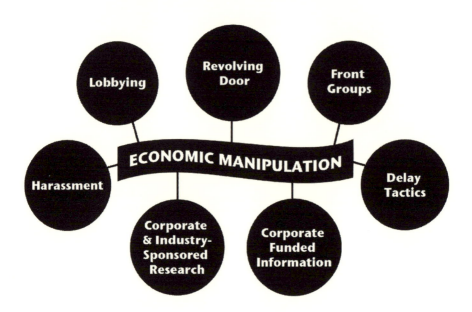

As of 2014, the controversy surrounding this synthetic substance has been an ongoing 44-year debate!

Aspartame, which is found in over 6,000 foods and beverages sold worldwide, is currently consumed by millions and millions of people *across the globe*. And to this day, although many shout from the rooftops that aspartame is absolutely safe, "Safety" has never actually been proven. A fact clearly shown by the numerous adverse reactions associated with aspartame consumption. That's why health advocates and medical experts around the world are still fighting to ban aspartame from the marketplace. Amazingly, some of these experts and advocates have dedicated nearly their entire careers to this one cause. And I sure appreciate their efforts.

So enough chatting; let's get on with it! But consider yourself warned...I found this to be pretty shocking stuff.

Discovery of Aspartame

Aspartame was discovered in 1965 when a G.D. Searle Co. chemist named James Schlatter was working on an ulcer drug. Legend has it that Schlatter serendipitously noticed the sweetness of aspartame when he licked his fingers after a bit of the mixture spilled out of the flask. Some say this story is ridiculous due to the fact that licking your fingers in a lab is a forbidden research practice, but that certainly doesn't mean it didn't happen.

Regardless of how aspartame was actually discovered, it was not made public until 1969.

Initial Approval: G.D. Searle, Lies, and Fraud

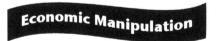

Economic Manipulation

On January 10, 1970, Searle approached Dr. Harry Waisman—a biochemist and respected expert in phenylalanine toxicity (phenylalanine is a main ingredient of aspartame)—to study the effects of aspartame on primates.[2]

In Waisman's study, seven infant monkeys were given milk with aspartame. After 300 days, one monkey died. Five others experienced grand mal seizures.[3-6] To say the very least, Dr. Waisman's results did not turn out too overly promising.

Interestingly, Dr. Waisman died unexpectedly in March 1971. Shortly thereafter, his study was terminated. Searle denied any knowledge of Waisman's study design, performance, or involvement therein.[2]

Around the same time, neuroscientist Dr. John Olney informed Searle that another main ingredient of aspartame—aspartic acid—caused holes in the brains of mice.[7] Dr. Olney also found that oral intake of aspartate (aspartic acid), glutamate (think MSG), and cysteine—all excitotoxic amino acids—caused brain damage in mice. However, Searle's representatives responded to Olney's findings by claiming that the data raised no health concerns.[3]

When Searle submitted its initial applications for aspartame approval, Dr. Waisman's disastrous results, as well as Dr. Olney's findings, were concealed from the FDA.[3-6]

The FDA Approves Aspartame

With aspartame's grievous test results and serious concerns hidden, the FDA accepted Searle's submitted studies. Even still, some of the

FDA's own officials felt Searle's studies were insufficient. One such official was Dr. Martha Freeman, FDA Division of Metabolic and Endocrine Drug Products.

After looking at Searle's submitted studies, Dr. Freeman concluded that "the information submitted for our review is inadequate to permit a scientific evaluation of clinical safety." She recommended that before marketing aspartame, the clinical safety of aspartame be proven.[5,8]

Of course, right? Safety should be demonstrated—beyond a shadow of a doubt—before unleashing a product on an unwitting public.

But that's not what happened.

The FDA Bureau of Foods, headed at that time by a man named Sherwin Gardner, ignored Dr. Freeman's suggestions. Instead, Gardner approved aspartame for limited use in foods on July 26, 1974. Approved uses of aspartame included as a sugar substitute for sweetening hot beverages, in cereals, gum, and dry bases.[9,10]

Why would Gardner do such a thing? We don't know for sure, however...

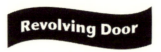

Revolving Door

FDA records show that Sherwin Gardner later resigned from his post as Deputy FDA Commissioner in 1979 to become a Vice President with Grocery Manufacturers of America (GMA), Inc.[11]

In case you don't know, GMA just happens to be the world's largest trade association for the food and beverage Industry. GMA lobbies, manages public relations, and directs political contributions for its member Corporations.

Though Mr. Gardner claimed that there was no conflict of interest, his employer (GMA) dealt directly with aspartame products.[11] GMA obviously greatly benefited from the approval of aspartame, and Gardner most likely received a substantial pay increase for overriding FDA officials' initial concerns.

> "The company laid out its strategy for getting aspartame approved by the FDA in a December 1970 [internal] memo. The goal: 'Bring [FDA officials] into a subconscious spirit of participation with Searle.'"[8]
>
> How did Searle plan to accomplish this? Psychology. By creating an "affirmative atmosphere" and coaxing FDA officials into the "habit of saying yes."[8]

THE SEARLE INVESTIGATIONS COMMENCE

By the time the FDA finally admitted the possibility of Searle's falsified and undisclosed test results surrounding aspartame, Searle's integrity was already in question. Serious side effects from a handful of their pharmaceutical drugs were beginning to surface, and the results of hundreds of other Searle studies were now deemed suspicious. Red flags were flying.

1975: FDA Special Task Force: The First Investigation

As a result of mounting suspicions, the reigning FDA Commissioner, Dr. Alexander Schmidt, appointed a special Task Force to investigate Searle in July 1975. The head of the Task Force was FDA Lead Investigator, Philip Brodsky, assisted by FDA Toxicologist, Dr. Adrian Gross.

The Task Force's job was to examine the quality and validity of Searle's safety testing practices by examining 25 key studies for the drugs Flagyl, Aldactone, Norpace, and the food additive aspartame. Eleven of these "pivotal" studies involved aspartame.

The Task Force was especially interested in "pivotal" tests for reasons described in a later article by Florence Graves in *Common Cause Magazine:*

"'Pivotal' tests include long-term (two-year) tests such as those done to determine whether aspartame might cause cancer. Former FDA commissioner Alexander Schmidt said in a recent interview that **if a pivotal test is found to be unreliable, it must be repeated** 'Some studies are more important than others, and **they have to be done impeccably,'** Schmidt said."[5,8]

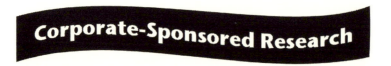

Corporate-Sponsored Research

Turns out, eighty percent of the "pivotal" tests conducted in the early 1970s were carried out either by Searle itself or by its main contractor, Hazleton Laboratories, Inc.[5,8]

What Did the 1975 FDA Task Force Conclude from Their Investigation of These Pivotal Studies?

Lo and behold, the Task Force found Searle's submitted studies unacceptable. They concluded that Searle's deliberate misconduct and "lies"—as put by FDA Investigator, Dr. Adrian Gross—invalidated their "research."[8]

Here are some highlights of the Task Force's conclusions, as stated in the Congressional Record 1985a:[8]

- "There were very serious deficiencies in Searle's operations and testing practices between 1967 and 1975... which undermine the reliance on Searle's integrity in conducting high-quality animal research to accurately determine or characterize the toxic potential of its products."

- The FDA Commissioner, Alexander Schmidt stated "[Searle's studies were] incredibly sloppy science. What we discovered was reprehensible."

- FDA Lead Investigator and Task Force Team Leader, Phillip Brodsky, who is described in the Task Force report as "one of the FDA's most experienced drug investigators," stated that he "had never seen anything" as "bad" as G.D. Searle's studies.

STATEMENT BY DR. ADRIAN GROSS, THE FDA TOXICOLOGIST:

"At the heart of FDA's regulatory process is its ability to rely upon the integrity of the basic safety data submitted by sponsors of regulated products. Our investigation clearly demonstrates that, in the (case of the) GD Searle Company, we have no basis for such reliance now.

We have noted that Searle has not submitted all the facts of experiments to FDA, retaining unto itself the unpermitted option of filtering, interpreting, and not submitting information which we would consider material to the safety evaluation of the product . . .

Finally, we have found instances of irrelevant or unproductive animal research where experiments have been poorly conceived, carelessly executed, or inaccurately analyzed or reported.

Some of our findings suggest an attitude of disregard for FDA's mission of protection of the public health by selectively reporting the results of studies in a manner which allay the concerns of questions of an FDA reviewer."[12]

What Did the 1975 Task Force Specifically Find That Led to Their Stated Conclusions?

"The extensive nature of the almost unbelievable range of abuses discovered by the FDA on several major Searle products is profoundly disturbing."
—*SENATOR EDWARD KENNEDY, UNITED STATES SENATE HEARINGS*[13]

Remember when I said this story was full of shocking stuff? Well, here we go...and these are just the highlights. This is a consummate example of what can—and obviously does—happen when Corporations/Industries are in charge of sponsoring their own research. The Task Force's preliminary investigations revealed that Searle's safety studies included, as Senator Kennedy stated in the quote above, "profoundly disturbing" practices, such as:[14-16]

- "Excising masses (tumors) from live animals, in some cases without histologic [studying tissues under a microscope] examination of the masses, without reporting them to the FDA."

  Astoundingly, when questioned about these actions, Searle's representatives stated that "these masses were in the head and neck areas and prevented the animals from feeding."

- "Failure to report to the FDA all internal tumors present in the experimental rats, e.g., polyps in the uterus, ovary neoplasms as well as other lesions."

- G.D. Searle "stored animal tissues in formaldehyde for so long that they deteriorated."

- "Instead of performing autopsies on rhesus monkeys that suffered seizures after being fed aspartame, the company had financed a new monkey seizure study with a different methodology that showed no problems."

- [There were] "clerical or arithmetic errors which resulted in reports of fewer tumors."

- [G.D. Searle] "delayed the reporting of alarming findings."

- "Selecting statistical procedures which used a total number of animals as the denominator when only a portion of the animals were examined, thus reducing the significance of adverse effects."

- "Presenting information to FDA in a manner likely to obscure problems, such as editing the report of a consulting pathologist . . . Reporting one pathology report while failing to submit, or make reference to another usually more adverse pathology report on the same slide."

Shocked yet??

The Result of the 1975 Investigation

Due to these preliminary findings of the FDA Task Force, the FDA put a hold on aspartame approval on December 5, 1975.

After completing their investigation, the FDA Task Force completed *a 500-page report with 15,000 pages of exhibits* and submitted it to the FDA in March 1976.

You'd think that would be enough to stop everything in its tracks, right?

Yeah, you'd think. But no.

1976 FDA Task Force—Jerome Bressler Leads the Second *Investigation*

In July 1976, the FDA launched another investigation to further examine three key aspartame studies in which the 1975 FDA Task Force discovered serious issues. This second Task Force was headed by FDA veteran Inspector, Jerome Bressler. The results of this investigation, which were revealed in 1977, became famously known as *The Bressler Report*. We'll see what kind of monkey business this investigation unearthed shortly.

In the meantime…

During Investigations, FDA Allows Searle to Hire UAREP, a Private Research Team

Corporate-Sponsored Research

Unbelievably, in August 1976, right in the midst of the *Bressler* investigation, the FDA permitted Searle to pay a private agency (known as UAREP) $500,000 to "validate" the other 12 studies examined by the 1975 Task Force, but not currently under investigation by Bressler.[16]

UAREP's (Universities Associated for Research and Education in Pathology), **only** job was to make sure the studies were actually conducted. "The pathologists were specifically told that they were not to make a judgment about aspartame's safety or to look at the designs of the tests."[8]

You gotta wonder... what's the flippin' point? And why on Earth would Searle be allowed to *pay* for the "validation" of studies that were already decidedly disturbing and poorly executed? Who *cares* if they were actually conducted—they were fraudulent!

Perhaps even more disconcerting—this particular Corporate Sponsored "validation" conducted by UAREP was heavily leaned upon in following debates over the safety of aspartame.

All the While

Corporate-Sponsored Information

In an attempt to gain support for aspartame's safety claims, *The Journal of Toxicology and Environmental Health* published a series of poorly conducted, blemished studies funded by Searle in 1976.[17]

The associate editor of this scientific journal? Robert G. McConnell.[2] McConnell just happened to be the director of Searle's Department of Pathology and Toxicology, and was largely responsible for the poor quality of the preapproval studies that were investigated by the first task force in 1975. Sounds like maybe McConnell was trying to cover his keister *and* make a couple of extra bucks?

Besides McConnell, there were two other Searle-employed editors of the journal, Carl Mackerer and Thomas Tephly. Tephly was later responsible for conducting a series of terribly flawed blood measurements, which spanned over 15 years, in NutraSweet® (aspartame)-funded studies.[17]

Grand Jury Investigation of Searle is Requested

So now, amongst the second investigation led by Jerome Bressler, the UAREP arrangement, and the recently published Corporate-planted studies, a little more craziness was added to the chaos…

On January 10, 1977, FDA Chief Counsel, Richard Merrill requested that the United States Attorney convene a Grand Jury to investigate the obvious crimes of Searle and its Officers. In light of the original 1975 Task Force findings, the crime was specifically cited as "violations of the Federal Food, Drug, and Cosmetic Act, 21 U.S. C.331(e), and the False Reports to the Government Act, 18 U.S.C. 1001."[4]

Merrill cited two especially flagrant aspartame studies in his 33-page letter to U.S. Attorney, Samuel Skinner:[4]

- The 52-week toxicity study of infant monkeys by Dr. Waisman in 1970 in which Searle withheld key findings from the FDA. If you recall, one monkey died and five others experienced grand mal seizures from ingesting aspartame.

- A 46-week hamster study in which Searle took healthy blood from hamsters at the 2nd week but stated that blood was drawn at the 38th week. In reality, many of the hamsters that Searle claimed the blood was drawn from at the 38th week were already dead.[18]

Economic Manipulation

Richard Merrill also specifically called out Robert McConnell—the director of Searle's Department of Pathology and Toxicology and also the Associate Searle-Sponsored Editor of *The Journal of Toxicology and Environmental Health*—in his letter to U.S. Attorney Samuel Skinner regarding the convening of a grand jury.

But in an unbelievable turn of events, McConnell's attorney reported that his client was asked to take a three-year, paid sabbatical at $60,000 per year (plus a $15,000 bonus) because he was a "political liability!"[16]

SOOoooooo instead of indictment for criminal activity, McConnell gets sent on a paid vacation??! Whoa.

But McConnell was only one of the guilty players. So while the FDA investigations proceeded, Merrill's request for a grand jury investigation remained in process.

And then, in a bold, and what would certainly seem illegal, turn of events…

The Law Firm Representing Searle Solicits U.S. Attorney Skinner

On January 26, 1977, just after Merrill sent his letter to U.S. Attorney Skinner requesting a grand jury investigation, Sidley & Austin, the law firm representing Searle, called for a meeting with Skinner.[16,19]

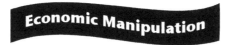

About six weeks later, on March 8, 1977, Skinner stated that he had begun preliminary employment discussions with Sidley & Austin. This statement appeared in a confidential memo to his aides, written while he was supposed to be working on fraud indictments against Searle.[16,19]

No conflict of interest here, right?

Then, on April 13, 1977, the U.S. Justice Department sent a memo to Skinner advising him to move forward with the grand jury investigations of Searle before the Statute of Limitations for prosecution expired. The expiration date for the Waisman study was October 10, 1977, and December 8, 1977 for the hamster study.[19]

Skinner withdrew from the case shortly thereafter, and Assistant U.S. Attorney William Conlon was assigned to take his place.[16] Their stories continue to unfold shortly.

But let's back up for a moment. Unfolding in the wings, right around the time the grand jury was requested, the revolving door had really begun to spin when…

Donald Rumsfeld Becomes Searle's President

Searle hired Rumsfeld to manage the aspartame approval issues as a "legal problem rather than a scientific problem."[16]
—CONSUMER ATTORNEY, JAMES TURNER

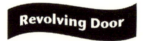

After completing his term, as White House Chief of Staff and then U.S. Secretary of Defense in the Gerald Ford Administration (September 1974 to January 1977), Donald Rumsfeld was hired by Searle in January 1977.[16]

He was allegedly hired for his "boy scout image" to mend fences with the FDA and pull Searle out of debt and controversy. To help accomplish this goal, Rumsfeld immediately hired three other outgoing Ford Administration officials to join him.[3]

Revolving Door   **Revolving Door**   **Revolving Door**

John Robson was hired as Searle's Executive Vice President. Robson had served as President Ford's chairman of the Civil Aeronautics Board (then connected to the Department of Transportation). Robson was also a former lawyer with Sidley & Austin, the law firm representing Searle.

Robert Shapiro, Robson's Special Assistant at the Transportation Department, was named General Counsel.

William Greener Jr. was appointed Searle's Chief Spokesman. Greener was a former spokesman in the Ford White House as well as Rumsfeld's Chief Spokesman at the Pentagon.

The Revolving Door Result:

The future of Searle pharmaceutical company
was now in the hands of lawyers and politicians.

🍃 THE REVOLVING RUMSFELD[20]

Rumsfeld had a long history in government, initially serving as a member of Congress, and then moving on to different positions throughout the Nixon administration before his term during the Ford administration. Under Ford, Rumsfeld served first as White House Chief of Staff and then U.S. Secretary of Defense.

After employment in Private Industry—most notably twelve years between Big Pharma and Biotech Industries—Rumsfeld returned to the White House under the Bush Administration as Secretary of Defense from January 2001 to December 2006.

As we will see, Rumsfeld is a consummate example of revolving door activity, using connections within private and public sectors to pull strings for people in high places, while making a very lucrative living doing so.

U.S. Attorneys, Skinner and Conlon are Seduced by The Dark Side

"Nothing at last is sacred but the integrity of your own mind."
—RALPH WALDO EMERSON

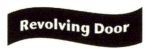

And the Revolving Door keeps spinning.

Disappointingly, on July 1, 1977, U.S. Attorney Samuel Skinner did indeed resign his post with the government to take a private position with Searle's law firm, Sidley & Austin.[16]

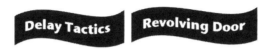

Doubly disappointing, although Assistant U.S. Attorney William Conlon (Skinner's successor) did manage to assemble a grand jury, he then proceeded to allow the Statute of Limitations to expire.[16]

Fifteen months later, Conlon followed his predecessor and also accepted a job with Sidley & Austin.[16]

HOW IS THIS LEGAL???

I dunno, but it sure as sh#$ shouldn't be!

And unfortunately, this plotting and scheming worked perfectly for Searle. The grand jury investigation was pronounced dead and a company that most definitely should have been severely penalized with criminal charges was off scot-free.

But wait, there's more…

The Bressler Report Results

In August 1977, the results of the second FDA investigation, headed by Jerome Bressler, were released. *The Bressler Report* revealed several more inexcusable research protocols, such as:[9, 19, 21-23]

- "One animal was reported alive at week 88, dead from week 92 through week 104, alive at week 108, and finally dead at week 112."

- "Tissue from some animals were noted to be unavailable for analysis on the pathology sheets, yet results from an analysis of this 'unavailable' tissue was submitted to the FDA."

- "There was evidence that the diet mix was not homogeneous, allowing the animals to eat around the test substance [aspartame ingredients]. This evidence included a picture and statements by a lab technician."

- "Fifteen fetuses from animals in one experiment were missing."

- "Sections from the animals were too thick for examination."

- "Animals were not permanently tagged to prevent mix-ups."

"THE QUESTION YOU HAVE GOT TO ASK YOURSELF:

Because of the importance of this study, why wasn't greater care taken? The study is highly questionable because of our findings.

Why didn't Searle, with their scientists, closely evaluate this, knowing fully well that the whole society, from the youngest to the elderly, from the sick to the un-sick . . . will have access to this product?"[16]

—Jerome Bressler

1978 Task Force: The Third *Investigation—Review of* The Bressler Report

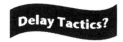

A review of an investigation of an investigation? When both investigations already clearly validated the reality of highly fraudulent research *and* continued to reveal more dirt?! Geesh! If there was so much controversy, and they weren't going to slam Searle with a felony, why didn't the FDA just trash the old studies and require completely new studies to be conducted by independent researchers?

That's the question. But we know the answer. And instead…

In 1978, immediately after the *Bressler Report* was released, the Director of FDA Bureau of Foods, H.R. Roberts, created another five-person task force to review the *Bressler Report*.

The review was conducted by a team at the Center for Food Safety and Applied Nutrition (CFSAN; the FDA division responsible for evaluating the safety of food additives.). Dr. Jacqueline Verrett, an FDA toxicologist, was appointed the senior scientist.

Dr. Verrett not only confirmed the results of the *Bressler* investigation, she had a couple of things to add. She was particularly concerned about a key study on the aspartame metabolite (byproduct) Diketopiperazine (DKP) and cancer.

In a testimony before the U.S. Senate, Dr. Verrett stated the following:[21]

- "There was no protocol written until the study was well underway."

  (Which basically means that they were making up the rules as they went along, most likely to control the outcome of the results.)

- "In some cases, tumors were removed, and the animals then returned to the study."

- "Of extreme importance is that in the DKP study there was evidence, including pictures found in notebooks at Searle, that the diets were not homogeneous [as cited in the *Bressler Report*], and that the animals could discriminate between feed and the included particles of DKP. In other words, they may or may not have been eating what it was assumed they were eating."

During this same testimony, Dr. Verrett also stated the following conclusions from the review:

- "In numerous instances, a definitive answer could not be arrived at because of the basic inadequacies and improper procedures used in the execution of these studies."

- "I would like to emphasize the point that we were specifically instructed not to be concerned with, or to comment upon, the overall validity of the study. This was to be done in a subsequent review [known as "The Public Board of Inquiry"], carried out at a higher level."

- "It would appear that the safety of aspartame and its breakdown products has still not been satisfactorily determined…"

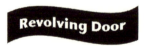

AFTER DR. VERRETT LEFT THE FDA, SHE OPENLY DISCUSSED THE 1978 TASK FORCE WITH INVESTIGATIVE REPORTER, GREGORY GORDON:

"Members were barred from stating opinions about the research quality. *'It seemed pretty obvious that somewhere along that line they (bureau officials) were working up to a whitewash,'* she said.

'I seriously thought of just walking off of that task force.' Verrett said that she and other members wanted to *'just come out and say that this whole experiment was a disaster and should be disregarded.'* "[16]

The Revolving Role of H.R. Roberts, FDA Bureau of Foods

In a submittal to FDA Dockets, Mark Gold of *the Aspartame Toxicity Information Center* stated that "It seemed that no matter how serious the mistakes were, the FDA Bureau of Foods was determined to accept the studies by G.D. Searle."[2]

Revolving Door

In fact, for each major issue outlined in the *Bressler Report*, the FDA Bureau of Foods Report had a comment to downplay the issue. Could this possibly be because H.R. Roberts, the Director of the FDA Bureau of Foods (November 1975 to October 1978), would leave his government role at the FDA to immediately become Vice President of

Science and Technology for the National Soft Drink Association in October 1978?[11]

In case you are not aware, aspartame is a key artificial sweetener in some of the largest brands of diet soft drinks.

So, no mystery here. And, yet again, certainly no conflict of interest, right?

Results of the Searle-Hired-UAREP "Research" Team

Corporate-Sponsored Research

UAREP submitted its *validation* of Searle's 12 aspartame studies on December 13, 1978. Not surprisingly, the UAREP report stated that there were "no discrepancies in any of the sponsor's reports that were of sufficient magnitude or nature that would compromise that data originally submitted."[9]

Well, c'mon, of course the findings were completely biased in favor of Searle. How would UAREP come to anything *but* a favorable conclusion when they were paid $500,000 to complete their review by a company being investigated for fraud?

And later, it was indeed discovered that UAREP pathologists completely failed to spot and/or withheld negative findings from the

FDA.[24] For example, when analyzing slides, there were studies wherein UAREP pathologists completely missed cancerous brain tumors. In another study, 12 animals actually had cancerous brain tumors, but UAREP reported that only three animals had such tumors. Furthermore, some of the slides to be inspected by UAREP pathologists were missing even though they were supposedly kept under "FDA seal."[25]

And the fact that *any* tumors were discovered and this product approval was not pulled *forever* is hard to imagine. How is that, in any way, okay?

However, unfathomably, these discoveries didn't stop officials from using the UAREP investigation as proof of aspartame's safety.[25]

"The notion that an industrial company would take large sums of money and parcel it out to scientific consulting firms and university departments, who they consider to be personal and commercial allies is an unconscionable way to ensure the safety of the American food supply."[16]
—*CONSUMER ATTORNEY TURNER*

AFTER ALL THAT... THE FDA ACTUALLY CONCLUDED THAT SEARLE'S STUDIES WERE ACCEPTABLE

Yep, believe or not, despite the repeated investigations into Searle's safety studies, which consistently found fraudulent data hiding the presence of tumors, seizures, and even death—all contained within piss-poor lab practices—the FDA (leaning heavily on the results of the UAREP "study") reached the conclusion that Searle's aspartame studies were valid.[2] WOW!

But, there was still one more chance to stop aspartame from hitting the market. The FDA finally decided to convene the Public Board of Inquiry (PBOI), which was agreed to four years earlier at the request of Dr. John Olney and Consumer Attorney James Turner.[26] Since Searle's studies were now considered "valid," the PBOI's job was to answer the question of whether or not aspartame should be allowed for use in foods. From the get-go, Dr. Olney (due to his own preliminary findings) and Attorney Turner had strong objections to the approval of aspartame and desperately pleaded for their concerns to be heard and taken seriously.

In a letter to Consumer Attorney, James Turner, the FDA general counsel responded to Mr. Turner's concerns about the quality and validity of Searle's studies. The FDA stated, "The Public Board of Inquiry on aspartame should provide a vehicle for definitive resolution, at least for those studies about which you are most concerned."[5,8]

THE LAST CHANCE TO STOP APPROVAL: THE PUBLIC BOARD OF INQUIRY (PBOI)

The PBOI was to be a three-person panel. Dr. John Olney, G.D. Searle, and the FDA's Bureau of Foods were all permitted to nominate potential panel scientists.[27]

> Searle is given yet *another* opportunity to
> choose their advocate? Blasphemy!
>
> Can you say...

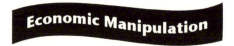

The Scope of the PBOI

This panel was strictly advised that there was to be no discussion about the validity of the pre-approval studies. This was now a closed question answered by UAREP as far as FDA officials were concerned. These members were instructed to simply accept the FDA's word that the studies were now considered "validated."[5,8]

In fact, the FDA restricted PBOI's scope to the following questions:[27]

- Does the ingestion of aspartame, either alone or together with glutamate, pose a risk of contributing to mental retardation, brain damage, or undesirable effects on the neuroendocrine system?

  By the way, "neuroendocrine" may as well read "nearly every single function in the human body!" No joke.

- May the ingestion of aspartame induce brain tumors in the rat?

And then based on the answers to those questions:

> ✓ Should aspartame be allowed for use in foods, or should approval of aspartame be withdrawn?

> ✓ If the approval for aspartame is not withdrawn, and it is allowed for use in foods, what are the conditions of use and should any labeling statements be required?

▼ OF EXTREME IMPORTANCE:

The PBOI—along with all of the other investigators on previous review boards—was only to consider aspartame for the use in dry goods, **not beverages!**

The PBOI Decision

In 1980, the Public Board of Inquiry voted and *unanimously* rejected the use of aspartame until additional studies on aspartame's potential to cause brain tumors were completed.[2]

THE PBOI REVOKED THE 1974 ASPARTAME APPROVAL.

YAY! Victory at last!! Justice is served.

But it didn't last long.

PRESIDENT REAGAN TAKES OFFICE AND SEARLE REAPPLIES FOR APPROVAL

Relentlessly, Searle reapplied for the approval of aspartame on January 21, 1981, the day after Ronald Reagan took office.[2] This was probably no mistake. In fact, it was suspected to be perfectly planned timing.[16]

Indeed, one might argue that all of these delays, and investigations-of-investigations-of–reviews-of-inquiries, were deliberately drawn out to coincide with Reagan's election. G.D. Searle's president was Donald Rumsfeld, after all, who had extremely tight and longstanding connections with the Elephant Party.

Apparently, Rumsfeld told his Searle sales force that "he would call in all his markers and that no matter what, he would see to it that aspartame would be approved that year," according to Patty Wood-Allott, former Searle salesperson.[16]

Toward that end, there was rumor that Reagan would be replacing Jere Goyan, the FDA Commissioner. Why? Apparently, "Rumsfeld was concerned that he [Goyan] would not approve aspartame because of his position on cyclamate."[28]

 ### FDA COMMISSIONER, JERE GOYAN, AND CYCLAMATE[29]

Cyclamate is an artificial sweetener that was banned for sale in the U.S. in October 1969.

Studies submitted by Abbott Laboratories did not demonstrate "to a reasonable certainty" that cyclamate was safe for human consumption.

Abbott Labs petitioned the FDA to lift the ban on cyclamate in 1973, and the petition was finally denied by FDA Commissioner Jere E. Goyan in September 1980.

His decision confirmed an earlier ruling by an administrative judge that the safety of cyclamate had not been demonstrated.

Interestingly, when I first began research on this topic, the FDA's status list stated that cyclamate was "held in abeyance" (suspension). However, now, interestingly enough, cyclamate status reads "illegal in food."[30]

Commissioner Goyan Calls Panel to Review Issues Raised by the PBOI

In March of 1981, FDA Commissioner Goyan launched yet another five-member panel of scientists to further review questions of concern raised by the PBOI regarding aspartame and potential neurotoxicity.[16,19]

It seems odd that Goyan would call yet another review, but perhaps it was necessary in order to put the issue to rest for good, while he was in charge. He clearly had plans to do the right thing because…

"Meanwhile President Reagan, as a favor to Rumsfeld, had the FDA Commissioner, [that was] about to sign the revoked petition into law, fired at 3:00 AM. He then wrote an executive order making the FDA powerless to do anything about aspartame until he could get Arthur Hull Hayes, a friend of Rumsfeld, appointed as FDA Commissioner to overrule the Board of Inquiry."
—*FROM DR. WOODROW MONTE'S, "WHILE SCIENCE SLEEPS"[31]*

As presumed, President Reagan appointed Arthur Hull Hayes, Jr., the new FDA Commissioner, in April 1981.[5,8]

PBOI Concerns Are Confirmed

On May 18, 1981, three of the scientists in this new five-member panel sent a letter to Joseph Levitt, the panel lawyer, outlining their concerns about aspartame.[16] Those three scientists were Satva Dubey (FDA Chief of Statistical Evaluation Branch), Douglas Park (FDA Staff Science Advisor), and Robert Condon (FDA Veterinary Medicine).

Dubey said that key data appeared to have been altered, and the brain tumor data was so "worrisome" that he could not advocate the approval of aspartame.[16]

In his UPI (United Press International) Investigation of the approval of aspartame, apparently the most thorough investigation ever completed, Gregory Gordon describes the unusual events that followed:[16,32]

- "Douglas Park said that [panel lawyer Joseph] Levitt hurried the panel to decide the issue. 'They wanted to have the results yesterday. We really didn't have the time to do the in-depth review we wanted to do.'"

- "Park said that Levitt met frequently with [Arthur Hull] Hayes and 'was obviously getting the pressure to get a resolution and a decision made.'"

- "With three of five scientists on the commissioner's team opposing approval, it was decided to bring in a toxicologist for his opinion on isolated issues [Barry N. Rosloff]."

    ✓ "Jere Goyan [Former FDA Commissioner] said if the decision were his, he never would have enlarged the team."

    ✓ "Levitt, who normally would have been expected to draft an options paper spelling out scientific evidence on key issues, took an unusual tack. He circulated *an approval recommendation* (emphasis is mine). Levitt said he was not directed to draft the approval memo, but did so as a 'tactical' step to break the team's weeks-long impasse by forcing each scientist to state his views." The decision to oppose approval ended up split right down the middle 3-3.

This was a tragic outcome. Had the five-member team been left to make the decision, it was clear that three of the five were against the approval of aspartame. By adding another member, Hayes and Levitt were able to finagle the outcome. And that is exactly what they did.

Economic Manipulation

Levitt was later promoted to a post as an executive assistant to the FDA Commissioner.[16,32]

HAYES BREAKS THE LAW TO APPROVE ASPARTAME

Yep, that's right. More illegal activity!

Arthur Hull Hayes Jr. overruled the Public Board of Inquiry and ignored the law—Section 409 (c)(3) of the Food Drug and Cosmetic Act (21 U.S.C. 348)—which declares that a food additive should not be approved if tests are inconclusive.[9,27]

On July 18, 1981, Hayes officially approved aspartame for use in dry foods.

And THEN…

An Amendment Is Created *to Extend Searle's Patent on Aspartame*

Due to all of the delays with investigations into the horrendous research studies on aspartame's safety, Searle's patent on the additive was about to expire.

You'd think… too bad, so sad… right?

However, on October 1, 1982, an obscure amendment was attached to the *Orphan Drug Act* (intended to encourage the development of new drugs for rare diseases).[33] This amendment extended the U.S. Patent law, but **only applied to** one product and one company—**aspartame and Searle.**[16]

Without direct mention of aspartame or Searle in legal documents, the senate passed the amendment. Searle's patent was extended by almost six years.[16]

Economic Manipulation

How did they pull this one off? Well, according to records, the officials involved in molding this amendment to fit Searle's needs received some financial incentive. For example:[16-32]

- Senator Howell Heflin, who proposed the amendment, received $9,000 from Searle's top officers and its political action committee.

- Senator Robert Byrd, who brought the amendment up for vote, received $1,000 from the CEO of Searle.

- The amendment was 'pushed through' by Representatives Henry Waxman and Orrin Hatch.

   - ✓ Representative Waxman received $1,500 from the soft drink political action committee.

   - ✓ Senator Hatch received $2,500 from the soft drink political action committee. Daniel Searle, Wesley Dixon (Daniel Searle's brother-in-law), and William Searle each gave Hatch $1,000 as well.

As we will see, Senator Hatch also played an instrumental role in repeatedly blocking later hearings in the continued battle to address aspartame's safety.

FDA'S OWN SAFETY STANDARDS IGNORED AGAIN AND ASPARTAME IS APPROVED FOR USE IN BEVERAGES

Although aspartame was only intended for use in dry foods (you'll see why shortly), aspartame was spontaneously approved for use in carbonated beverages and carbonated beverage syrup bases in 1983.[34]

The approval was signed by Mark Novitch, who was standing in for FDA Commissioner Arthur Hull Hayes while out of town. I'm sure, for whatever reason, this was no mistake in their world of highly calculated actions. Of course, Hayes worked closely with Novitch on this issue.[16]

With their approval for use in beverages, Novitch and Hayes disregarded the FDA's own safety standards regarding the Acceptable Daily Intake (ADI) of aspartame. I'm not sure how they even determined an ADI without proving the safety of aspartame in the first place. In any case, with aspartame now allowed in beverages, CFSAN (FDA's food additive division) conveniently and spontaneously decided it was safe to more than double the ADI from 20 mg/kg to 50 mg/kg.[11,35]

The financial results of Hayes's approval for aspartame use in beverages were obviously HUGE for Searle. Searle's U.S. sales of Aspartame and Equal® reached $74 mil in 1982 before it was used in beverages. By the end of 1983, sales reached an astronomical $336 million, as a result of aspartame use in carbonated beverages.[8]

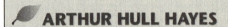 **ARTHUR HULL HAYES**

Shortly after the FDA approval for aspartame in carbonated beverages, FDA Commissioner Hayes apparently left the FDA in September 1983 on charges of "improprieties." Impropriety is a very far-reaching word that could refer to anything from using foul language to engaging in corruption. So that tells us very little.

Regardless, it appears there were no bona fide consequences for Hayes's criminal behavior. In fact, after leaving his government post at the FDA, Hayes was hired by Burson Marsteller, Searle's public relations firm, as a consultant at $1,000/day in November of that same year.[16,32]

Approval Objections and Requests For Hearings Are Denied

In July 1983, both Dr. Woodrow Monte, Director of the Science and Nutrition Laboratory at Arizona State University, and Consumer Attorney James Turner filed petitions objecting to the approval of aspartame.

The FDA denied requests to hold aspartame's approval "because public interest did not require it," while also denying Dr. Monte and Turner the opportunity to hold a hearing to address the questions outlined in their petitions.[36]

Dr. Monte was particularly concerned with the chronic intake of methanol from aspartame consumption. To address that concern, he also filed a petition with the Arizona Department of Health Services to hold a hearing to discuss a ban on aspartame.[16]

Decomposition Issues Raised By the State of Arizona and the National Soft Drink Association (NSDA)

Along with approval for use in beverages, came yet another safety issue.

In 1984, The Arizona Department of Health Services completed research showing that when exposed to high temperatures (beginning around 86°F), the aspartame in carbonated beverages could in fact break down into free methanol (we'll learn more about the danger of this shortly). The findings concerned the DHS enough to discuss Dr. Monte's suggestion for a ban on aspartame.[16,32]

The Congressional Report 1985a also confirms the decomposition issues, stating that a soft drink could frequently be exposed to temperatures between anywhere from 90°F to 151°F (whether in southern states in the summer, a car parked in the sun, or sitting in an ambient warehouse).[8]

Even Searle's own studies stated that aspartame's rate of degradation was directly connected to PH and temperature, noting that "as temp increases, the rate of degradation becomes more pronounced."[8] Furthermore, the degradation occurred in a short period of time.

Of course, Searle never demonstrated that aspartame was safe to consume in beverages under specific time and temperature conditions. How could they? Searle never proved aspartame was safe under *any* condition. In fact, the Congressional Report 1985a states that "Searle has not met its burden of proof under section 409 (cX3XB) of the FDC Act. 21 U.S.C. 348 (cX3XB)."[8]

Even the National Soft Drink Association (NSDA) expressed concern about the breakdown of aspartame when exposed to high heat, stating that aspartame is fundamentally unstable.[8] Later, however, the NSDA mysteriously dismissed their concerns without any explanation. Theory says the NSDA wielded this information not because they were worried about public safety, but to negotiate a lower buying price for aspartame.[8]

The State of Arizona Is Bought Off

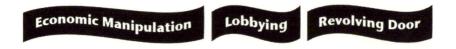

The State of Arizona's concerns about aspartame's toxicity were apparently assuaged with campaign contributions, along with lobbyists gifting whatever was necessary to buy off their worries. For example:

- Searle officials contributed to Burton Barr, Arizona House Majority Leader, between August and September 1984.[16,32]

- Later, Barr's Reelection Committee gave contributions to a number of state representatives (Don Aldridge, Karen Miills, Jan Breuer), all of whom eventually voted in favor of Searle.[16,32]

- Also in 1984, Searle sent several lobbyists to the State of Arizona, including a former Arizona Governor Chief of Staff, a Searle lawyer, a Searle official, and a high-flying Arizona lobbyist named Charles Pine.[3,16,32]

🍃 UP CLOSE:

Gregory Gordon's UPI investigation revealed that Searle hired up to a dozen lobbyists and gave around $200,000 in federal campaign contributions between 1973 and 1986 from its officers and political action committee.[16]

And that's just what was in the records.

And then…the Arizona legislature pulled a sneaky maneuver. They eliminated the text in a Toxic Waste Bill and then used it to pass another bill that prohibited regulation of FDA-approved food additives.[16,32] Who knows how, but that's what happened.

As a result, the outright concerns about degradation were seemingly forgotten. Dr. Monte's suggestions regarding discussion for a ban on aspartame were dismissed. And Searle ended up winning… again.

But the battle for justice continued to march on as…

Senator Howard Metzenbaum Fights for Labeling

Quantity consumption (acceptable daily intake or ADI) is a key component raised by worried scientists regarding whether aspartame is indeed safe to consume, or not. One of the ensuing concerns is that, without labeling, a person cannot possibly determine the quantity of aspartame they are consuming.

Toward that end, on May 7, 1985, Senator Howard Metzenbaum presented an amendment that would require a product to label the quantity of aspartame it contained. The U.S. Senate heard the testimony.[8]

Senator Hatch stepped in to lead the fight against the labeling amendment alongside Searle. Not surprisingly, the amendment was defeated.

On August 1, 1985, Senator Metzenbaum made another attempt at labeling and introduced a bill called the "Aspartame Safety Act of 1985." This bill took the previous amendment one step further and included a mandated moratorium on novel uses of aspartame until independent tests were conducted. The bill was submitted to a Senate committee, where sadly, it died.[35]

"I don't know of any company that has apparently covered all of its bases as well as has Searle," said Sen. Metzenbaum (D-Ohio). "Whether it has to do with the scientists or lawyers, or non-profit

institutions, or universities, or whatever; in every instance, I have found that they have expended their dollars very carefully and very wisely, but without apparent restraint as to the amount."[16]

MONSANTO BUYS G.D. SEARLE CO. AND RUMSFELD CLEANS UP

Monsanto, the ubiquitous chemical giant, bought G.D. Searle in 1985 for about $2.7 billion cash.[37] With this acquisition, the NutraSweet Company was born, created by Monsanto, as a wholly owned subsidiary of Searle.[32]

As a result, after nine years as Searle's President—and the leader of the successful turnaround—Revolving-Door-Rumsfeld left in solid financial condition. It's challenging to pin down the exact figure, but Rumsfeld appears to have earned around $12 million when Searle sold to Monsanto.[38]

Furthermore, although I couldn't find actual documentation of his salary, many claim that Securities and Exchange Commission records show that, between 1979 and 1984, Rumsfeld earned more than $2 million in salaries and more than $1.5 million in bonuses for guiding Searle to success. No small change, especially in the early '80s.

ASPARTAME OPPONENT LOSES FUNDING FOR INDEPENDENT RESEARCH

Harassment

Dr. Richard Wurtman of MIT, a former Searle consultant, quit his job and became a NutraSweet opponent after he recognized the danger of aspartame.

Dr. Gerald Gaull, then Searle Vice President, paid a visit to Dr. Wurtman's lab in 1985 and threatened to veto his funding from the International Life Sciences Institute (a Washington D.C. based lobby group funded by food, chemical, and drug companies)[39] if he continued on with his intended study on aspartame, brain chemistry, and human seizure thresholds. Dr. Wurtman did not discontinue his research and his funding was indeed withdrawn.[2, 32]

Interestingly enough, Dr. Wurtman later became silent and pulled his book, "*Dietary Phenylalanine and Brain Function,*" from the shelves.[40] Although we're not exactly sure why he disengaged, it isn't too hard to take an educated guess.

ASPARTAME CONSUMPTION SKYROCKETS

In 1984, 6,900,000 pounds of aspartame were consumed in the U.S. By 1987, consumption climbed to an estimated 17,100,000 pounds.[41] That's almost a 250% increase in sales in just three years, and those figures are solely for the U.S.! Aspartame has slithered into markets all across the globe in efforts to build what is termed "diet segments" to increase sales.[2]

After 1987, NutraSweet stopped providing consumption data to the USDA, perhaps because "it is much easier for NutraSweet scientists to create inaccurate aspartame consumption figures when the total number of pounds sold is not publically available."[2]

THE GOVERNMENT ACCOUNTING OFFICE LEADS A FINAL INVESTIGATION

Bless his heart, Senator Metzenbaum continued to fight the aspartame racket, and requested that the U.S. Government Accounting Office (GAO) review the FDA's approval process, including conflicts of interest.[42]

And the GAO did in fact conduct a review.

 WHAT IS THE ROLE OF THE GAO?[43]

"GAO's role is to support the Congress in carrying out its constitutional responsibilities and to help improve the performance and assure accountability of government for the benefit of the American people."

One of the fundamental ways it carries out its mission:

"Oversight–**preventing and detecting fraud, waste, abuse, and mis-management.**"

With a mission statement like the GAO's, you'd think: finally, at last, at least some of the FDA officials would be seen as guilty, and the approval process would be seen as at least suspicious, right?

Yes, of course. In an ideal world, that is.

But in June 1987, the GAO published the following conclusions from their reviews: [9,42]

- "FDA adequately followed its food additive approval process in approving aspartame for marketing by reviewing all of Searle's aspartame studies, holding a public board of inquiry to discuss safety issues surrounding aspartame's approval, and forming a panel to advise the Commissioner on those issues. Furthermore, when questions were raised about the Searle studies, FDA had an outside group of pathologists [Searle-hired-UAREP] review crucial aspartame studies."

- "Because FDA followed its required approval process in approving aspartame and monitors adverse reactions and ongoing aspartame research, GAO is making no recommendations."

But that's not all…

The author of the report specifically stated in the cover letter to Senator Metzenbaum on page one:

> "However, GAO did not evaluate the interpretation of the scientific issues raised or the adequacy of FDA's resolution of issues on the studies used for aspartame's approval, nor did it determine aspartame's safety; GAO does not have such expertise."

Can You Say *Worthless*?

Furthermore, with regard to conflicts of interest, the GAO glossed over, reworded, or completely overlooked key components such as:

- The revolving door activity of *many* key players involved in the approval process, as well as discussions of future employment, *while still in office*.

  I only covered some of the heavy hitters, but in October 1987, the United Press reported that *more than 10 federal officials involved in the approval of aspartame* took jobs in the private sector linked to the aspartame Industry. These officials included the Deputy FDA Commissioner, the Special Assistant to the FDA Commissioner, the Associate Director of the Bureau of Foods and Toxicology, and the Attorney involved with the Public Board of Inquiry.[3,16]

- The FDA allowing Searle to hire UAREP for $500,000 to "validate" their studies and then using the UAREP review as a fundamental argument for aspartame's safety, regardless of the issues that were later found with the review.

- The "whitewashed" evaluations, such as CFSAN's evaluation of the *Bressler Report*.

- The fact that the FDA Commissioner Hayes *illegally* approved aspartame against the advice of his own scientists. AND decided it was A-okay to use in beverages.

- Not to mention the various and vitally important flaws in the preapproval studies, and the severe reactions or fatal results suffered by animals in the studies.

I mean, c'mon... *R e a l l y??*

Like previous investigations, it seems the GAO was only *vaguely* paying attention to whether the FDA took the appropriate steps in a legal sense, and was not concerned with whether or not the FDA's decisions were in fact *legal,* rational, or based on accurate information.[2,24] And conflicts of interest were clearly ignored. I read the reports, which read like the crafty creation of wordsmiths. Twisting and turning key findings, concerns, and the slippery dealings of key officials—while taking their word for actions that necessitated further investigation—to suit the goals and desires of whoever was greasing their palms.

As you can see, a wide array of individuals, with a vested interest in Profit and Power, absolutely committed to a predetermined outcome, regardless of concerns surrounding public safety, can make the impossible, possible.

🍃 HOW IS THE REVOLVING DOOR *NOT* ILLEGAL?

The aspartame-approval-game is an exemplary example of how the "revolving door" allows large, powerful Corporations to gain control over government action and legislation.

Believe it or not, the revolving door is not an illegal activity per say, as the regulations do "not require **former** [but what about discussions while *still in office*?] government employees to decline employment with private organizations." However, "federal postemployment regulations do place certain restrictions on such employees' contacts with their former agencies."[11]

So with regard to the aspartame controversy, as far as I understand, the "certain restriction" simply meant that former FDA employees (now employed by private industry) could not return to the FDA *to discuss aspartame* if they had been involved in the approval process. At least not for a specified period of time, which was one to two years, depending upon the position they held at the FDA. The only restriction then, really, is that the former official cannot return to their government agency to discuss a product in which he/she was directly involved for a certain period of time. Period. These incredibly malleable guidelines leave waaaaayyy too much wiggle room for interpretation. And they could not—and obviously did not—cover all the multitudes of revolving door permutations that exist. Not to mention the conflicts of interest therein.

According to the GAO, this federal "postemployment statute" is intended "to preserve and promote public confidence in the integrity of federal officials through financial disclosure, postemployment restrictions, and independent investigations of alleged wrongdoing by government officials."[11] Hhhhhmmm. Interesting. So where is YOUR confidence level in the integrity of our federal officials right about now?

AND THE REST IS HISTORY

So even with fraudulent testing and blatantly illegal decisions—not to mention the very real possibility of brain tumors, brain damage, cancer, and the like—aspartame was approved and is still on the market today, leaving the public to be the daily lab rats.

Concerned medical experts, independent scientists, as well as citizens who have suffered from aspartame's effects, are still fighting, but aspartame-containing products continue to line the shelves of the grocery stores.

Now that we know how aspartame reached the market, let's take a look at what it's made of and how it affects people today.

WHAT EXACTLY IS ASPARTAME ANYWAY?

NOTE: Although I've simplified this to the best of my ability, this section may get a tiny bit techy for some people. Please hang with me, because the aspartame-is-safe folks are counting on your ignorance about the true nature of this artificial sweetener.

Aspartame, scientifically known as *aspartyl phenylalanine-methyl ester,* is a synthetic chemical that is approximately 180+ times sweeter than sugar. It is created by combining two amino acids (40% aspartic acid and 50% phenylalanine) and holding them together with a methyl ester bond (10% methanol). When aspartame is ingested, the methyl ester bond is broken, and aspartame breaks down into these three preliminary components: aspartic acid, phenylalanine, and methanol.

Proponents claim that aspartame is a "natural" substance because it contains amino acids—the building blocks of protein essential for nearly every bodily function. And while it is true that amino acids are absolutely vital for good health, the amino acids in aspartame are used in free-form, as an "isolate," meaning they are separated from their natural protein chain. These are *manufactured replicas* of the amino acids naturally found in our bodies and/or natural food sources. So don't be fooled. Aspartame is anything but natural. This compound is made in a lab, not nature.

And here is the crux of the concern with these lab-made amino acids:

When free-form amino acids are consumed, they enter the central nervous system in abnormally high concentrations, and excess amounts can be difficult for the body to process and tolerate.

The Skinny on the Basic Breakdown Components

ASPARTIC ACID

Aspartic acid is required for protein synthesis and detoxification of your bloodstream.

It is an important but *non-essential* amino acid, meaning it is made by your body and does not need to be consumed in your diet.

Aspartic acid is known as an *excitotoxin*. Excitotoxins are amino acids that also serve as neurotransmitters (chemical messengers that communicate information throughout your brain and body). In their natural form, in small amounts, excitotoxins are essential for proper brain function and communication.

However, when excitotoxins are present in abnormally high concentrations in the body—as with *free-form* aspartic acid—brain cells (neurons) and peripheral nerves (which conduct information to and from the central nervous system), become hyper-stimulated and begin to fire abnormally.

This unnaturally occurring excitation can create a breakdown of nerve function. And when concentrations become high enough, nerve cells can become so over-stimulated that they actually die. This excitatory process can amplify pain signals in the body, as well as create uncontrollable anxiety, irritability, and behavioral issues.

PHENYLALANINE

Phenylalanine is an *essential* amino acid, meaning it must be consumed in your diet because your body doesn't make it. Naturally occurring phenylalanine is found in most protein-containing foods such as beef, poultry, pork, fish, milk, yogurt, eggs, cheese, and soy products.

Phenylalanine is required for protein synthesis and to make brain chemicals, including L-dopa, epinephrine, norepinephrine, and thyroid hormones. Consequently, this amino acid is necessary for things like cognitive function and emotional well-being.

Like aspartic acid, the phenylalanine in aspartame is a "free-form" amino acid, and too much of it can cause a rapid increase in the levels of phenylalanine in the brain.

Phenylalanine isn't a health concern for most people, unless it builds up excessively in the body, specifically the brain. However, individuals with the genetic disorder phenylketonuria (PKU) cannot metabolize phenylalanine. As a consequence, ingestion can lead to dangerously high and sometimes lethal levels of phenylalanine in the brain. Phenylalanine can cause mental retardation, brain damage, seizures, and other problems in people with PKU. Luckily, newborns are routinely checked for PKU.

Apparently, phenylalanine can also trigger emotional and behavioral disorders in individuals who don't have PKU, but who take the following prescriptions or have the following conditions:

- Monoamine oxidase inhibitors, neuroleptics, or medications that contain levodopa
- Pregnant
- Tardive dyskinesia
- Sleep disorder
- Anxiety disorder or other mental health condition

If you relate to any of the above, please watch your phenylalanine consumption and/or talk to your doctor.

NOTE: Products that contain phenylalanine are required to be labeled as such.

METHANOL

Methanol is also known as methyl alcohol or wood alcohol. It is used for making substances such as formaldehyde, acetic acid, methyl t-butyl ether (a gasoline additive), paint strippers, carburetor cleaners, and chloromethanes.[44] Holy mackerel! Why on earth would methanol be used in anything we might *eat*?

Well, turns out, methanol is very sweet in small amounts, making it an attractive ingredient to use in artificial sweeteners. Methanol is also *naturally* found in overripe fruit, fruit juices, canned produce, fermented foods, and sometimes alcoholic beverages such as whiskey, wine, and beer.

Depending upon the source, methanol might be inhaled from vapors, absorbed through the skin, or ingested.

The Issue with Methanol Is Toxic Breakdown

Apparently, it's not so much the methanol itself in aspartame that poses a problem, but the toxic breakdown of methanol, which can be far more dangerous. When aspartame is consumed, most of the methanol is rapidly absorbed through the stomach where it's then converted into formaldehyde, a known carcinogen.[45,46]

But there are differing theories about what happens next. Animal studies say that our bodies further convert formaldehyde into formic acid,[44] and that formic acid is responsible for methanol poisoning.[47] However, according to aspartame expert Dr. Woodrow Monte, humans are the *only animal* lacking the key enzymes necessary to convert formaldehyde into formic acid, and so the culprit is indeed formaldehyde itself.[48-50]

Considering Dr. Monte has virtually dedicated his life to this topic, I have complete faith in his conclusion. But regardless of which conclusion is correct, the end result is clear: Ingesting too much methanol—and thus its breakdown products—is toxic to our bodies. In fact, according to the EPA, methanol is a "cumulative poison due to the low rate of excretion once it is absorbed by the human body."[51] This means, even small amounts of methanol from aspartame-containing products may accumulate over time, potentially causing health issues in the long run.[49]

The Establishment's Big Justification About Methanol in Aspartame

In 1984 the FDA stated that "no evidence" had established that the methanol byproduct reaches toxic levels, asserting that "many fruit juices contain higher levels of the natural compound."[52] Of course, pro-aspartame people concur: Methanol from aspartame is unlikely to be a safety concern, and consuming methanol from aspartame is *less* harmful than consuming naturally occurring methanol in fruits, fruit juices, and the like.

But that rationale simply isn't correct. Why? Because naturally occurring methanol is not the same as free methanol in aspartame.

Here are some of nature's protective mechanisms:

- Naturally occurring methanol in fresh fruit and vegetables is always accompanied by higher amounts of ethanol,[53] which acts as an antidote for methanol toxicity (ethanol is actually administered as a treatment for methanol poisoning).[54] Ethanol helps inhibit the metabolism of methanol, which allows the body to eliminate it before it converts to toxic byproducts.[55,56]

- Fresh fruits and other unprocessed foods also contain natural protective chemicals, which must also help prevent the methanol from converting to formaldehyde.[57] This does not include bottled, processed, canned, or commercial fruits, veggies, and juices that have been exposed to heat and lost their nutrients in processing.

- The methanol in fruit is bound to pectin, which can guide safe passage through your digestive tract.[58]

Common sense says that at least some of these factors, if not all, must come into play. Otherwise consumers of large quantities of fruits and vegetables, like myself, would surely be suffering from chronic methanol poisoning by now!

Made in a lab or made in nature… which do YOU trust?

So How Much Methanol Is Okay To Ingest?

There is a lot of controversy around the question of whether there is *enough* methanol in aspartame to harm the body.

The EPA's recommended limit of consumption for methanol is 7.8 mg per day, while it is estimated that most people consume up to 10 mg of methanol daily, as part of their regular diet.[51]

To put this in perspective, one 12-ounce can of aspartame-sweetened soda contains about 200 mg of aspartame, and 10% of this is methanol. So following digestion, you will add 20 mg of methanol to your diet. It is estimated that heavy consumers of aspartame-containing products may ingest up to 250 mg of methanol daily, which is over 32 times the EPA limit![51]

Remember, in the *Decomposition Issues Raised by the State of Arizona* section, we learned that free methanol is also created when aspartame is heated above 86°F? This can happen with prolonged storage or when an aspartame-containing product is heated, as in dessert mixes, gelatins, or a diet soda basking in the sunshine.

So, the question is…how can you possibly know how much methanol an aspartame product actually contains?

Suffice it to say, it's probably best not to consume too much methanol, especially in forms that do not contain naturally protective mechanisms. Like anything else, moderation is our safest solution.

🍃 TOO SCI-FI TO BE TRUE?

Can formaldehyde from methanol breakdown in aspartame lead to *PRE-EMBALMING?* EEEeekkkkkk!

The idea is discredited by some but highly cited by others. H. J. Roberts, M.D., addresses the issue of *pre-embalming* in his 1,000-page medical text, *Aspartame Disease: An Ignored Epidemic.*[59]

Roberts says:

"Inferences by funeral directors about the 'pre-embalming' of persons who had been heavy aspartame consumers initially evoked considerable skepticism.

But this theme kept surfacing. One experienced undertaker literally warned his family against using diet sodas after repeatedly detecting the deposition of formaldehyde crystals deposited in the organs of such individuals. Some funeral directors even insisted on closing the caskets of persons who had consumed large amounts of aspartame because formaldehyde seeped through the skin."

Whether you believe it or not, it does make you stop and think. Formaldehyde *is* embalming fluid after all.

ONE FINAL BYPRODUCT OF ASPARTAME: DIKETOPIPERAZINE (DKP)

Lastly, there is DKP, a 2% decomposition byproduct of aspartame, which has no sweetening properties. DKP is formed in liquid aspartame-containing products during prolonged storage, progressively degrading when exposed to temperatures ranging from 86° to 176°F.[60]

The concern among worried scientists is that DKP from aspartame might undergo a nitrosation (conversion) process in the stomach, producing a type of chemical that could cause brain tumors.[61,62]

The Acceptable Daily Intake (ADI) of diketopiperazine for humans has been established at 7.5 mg/kg body weight.[63]

Once again, I'm not sure how this figure is helpful, since the amount of DKP will be dependent upon storage time and temperature exposure. We have absolutely no way of knowing how much DKP may be present in an aspartame-containing product.

 DKP

"Not only is aspartame being used in the absence of basic toxicity information, but there is also no data to assess the toxicity of the interactions of DKP with the excess phenylalanine generated, with any other metabolite of aspartame, and its interactions with other additives, drugs, or other chemicals which may be present simultaneously in persons exposed to high levels of DKP in presweetened liquids such as diet drinks."

M. Jacqueline Verrett, Ph.D., former FDA toxicologist, in her testimony before Congress on November 3, 1987.[21]

I have two words for you:
Chemical Cocktail.

THE ASPARTAME MARKETING MACHINE

So tell me: Do YOU think aspartame is safe to consume?

We know the FDA does. In fact, the FDA argues that aspartame is one of the most tested food additives in U.S. history, with more than 100+ animal and human studies supporting its safety.[42]

Those studies do in fact exist, but remember to ask yourself:

Who conducted these studies and can you trust their results?

Corporate-Sponsored Research

In a *Survey of Aspartame Studies,* Dr. Ralph Walton reported:

"Of the 166 studies felt to have relevance for questions of human safety, 74 had NutraSweet® industry-related funding and 92 were independently funded. One hundred percent of the industry funded research attested to aspartame's safety, whereas 92% of the independently funded research identified a problem. Questions are raised both about aspartame's safety and the broader issue of the appropriateness of industry sponsorship of medical research."[64]

And, of course, there is loads and LOADS of...

Corporate-Sponsored Information

Obviously many Corporations rely on aspartame for their products, and as such, they churn out all kinds of encouraging information through an abundance of different channels. Whether found in peer-reviewed journals, front group propaganda, or non-profit literature, Corporate-Sponsored Aspartame Information is indeed rampant.

To add insult to injury, we must also remember that Monsanto manufactures aspartame—under the NutraSweet name—which donates its fair share of money to universities[65] and non-profit organizations,[66] while also employing PR and marketing firms to ensure their products sell.

Sell, sell, sell.

Coca-Cola and the American Cancer Society

Here is an interesting example worth noting: The Coca-Cola Company relies on aspartame for its widely consumed diet soda. So, as you might expect, their website touts the benefits of aspartame, while snubbing any hazards. A no-brainer, blatant conflict of interest, right? You bet.

However, what you might not expect—and therefore could throw you for a loop—is that Coca-Cola cites the American Cancer Society

(ACS) as proof that aspartame is safe.[67] Although ACS attempts to be somewhat diplomatic in their Q & A section on aspartame—using phrases like "in most cases" aspartame has not been linked to increased cancer risk in people—their green-light safety conclusion is clear.[68]

But guess what? Many of the American Cancer Society's heavy-hitting donors come directly from Big Food (including Coca-Cola, thank you very much), as well as Big Pharma, Big Chem, and even a hotshot law firm that represents these very Industries.[69] Consequently, ACS is the world's largest and wealthiest non-profit organization, allegedly holding over a billion dollars in cash.[70] So I wouldn't put too much stock in ACS literature, which can likely be bought, sold, or borrowed for the right price.

The Calorie Control Council

The *Calorie Control Council (CCC)* is one important-to-mention, ever-present example of a front group that vehemently rallies for aspartame.

As stated on its website:[71]

> The Calorie Control Council is an international, non-profit association "representing the low-calorie and reduced-fat food and beverage industry. Today it represents manufacturers and suppliers of low-calorie, low-fat and light foods and beverages, including the manufacturers and suppliers of more than two

dozen different alternative sweeteners, fibers and other low-calorie, dietary ingredients."

Ok, well that sounds pretty straightforward.

But who is really behind the CCC?

As stated by the CCC itself: "The Calorie Control Council is managed by the Kellen Company."[72]

So then, who is the Kellen Company?

As stated on their website: Kellen Communications "is a public relations agency" that provides a variety of services including advertising, branding development, social media, *crisis communication*, internet and search engine marketing, media relations, internet and search engine marketing, etc.[73]

"Our team includes seasoned public relations strategists, former journalists, experienced brand marketers, nutritionists, scientists and technical specialists, web developers, graphic designers, bloggers and governmental affairs professionals."[74]

"With the fragmentation of today's audiences, a communications program must use a variety of new media and traditional media tactics to reach targeted demographic audiences with clear, customized messages."[75]

Now with that information in mind—that a PR company is creating and managing the CCC websites—take a look at the websites copyrighted by the CCC:

- www.aspartametruth.org (*The Truth About Aspartame*)
- www.aspartameissafe.com
- www.aspartame.org

Amazing, huh?

I'm sure there are others, but these are the pro-aspartame sites connected to the CCC of which I am aware. It's not hard to figure out. If you scroll down to the bottom of the page, you'll see that the sites are indeed copyrighted by the *Calorie Control Council*, at least at the time of this writing. Remember that this kind of easy information could change as folks figure out that we are becoming more educated.

Easy-To-Spot Aspartame-Pushing Organizations

If you'd like to see an easy list of aspartame-pushing organizations that you would be wise to ignore—for any kind of dietary advice whatsoever, I might add—you can simply go directly to the horse's mouth: the NutraSweet website,[76] where you will see the following organizations listed:

- The European Food Information Council
- Grocery Manufacturers of America
- International Food Information Council (IFIC)
- International Sweeteners Association
- National Soft Drink Association (NSDA)

THE BOTTOM LINE

Any person or organization who receives funding or incentives from the aspartame Industry cannot be trusted as a source of accurate information! Always search for the sponsor.

WHAT'S THE REALITY BEHIND THE MARKETING?

In 1995, the FDA stated that 75% of the adverse reactions reported to the FDA Adverse Reaction Monitoring System (ARMS) were due to aspartame consumption.[57] The FDA reported receiving 7,000+ complaints of aspartame toxicity reactions up to that point.[77]

However, FDA officials also estimated that as little as 1% of the adverse reactions due to aspartame consumption were actually reported to the FDA,[78] most likely because the general public was not aware of ARMS (which only began in 1984). Furthermore, the FDA did not encourage physicians to report aspartame toxicity reactions;[79] only "serious" reactions were to be forwarded to FDA headquarters.[80] In addition, when people did call to report reactions to the FDA, there were numerous occasions when they were told that there was no association between adverse reactions and aspartame, and no further information was collected.[81]

So, based on the FDA's numbers, along with an estimated 1% reporting rate, a more realistic calculation of toxicity reactions would be closer to 700,000 *recognized* aspartame toxicity reactions in the

U.S. between 1982 and 1995.[77] However, this estimation does not include unrecognized and therefore unreported reactions—ranging from mild to serious illnesses—which would throw this calculation of toxicity reactions far into the *millions*.[57,77]

And how did the FDA respond?

In 1995, the FDA epidemiology branch chief was quoted as saying, "FDA has no further plans to continue to collect adverse reaction reports or monitor research periodically done on aspartame."[79]

Are you kidding me? How does *that* make any sense?

It doesn't, of course. So the reason for this decision had to rest on claims made by the FDA and NutraSweet Corporation that reports of adverse reactions had substantially decreased since the mid-1980s.[82,83]

In reality, the FDA continued to track reactions until at least 1997, as shown in records.[84] And at that time, there were over 10,000 filed complaints and 92 documented symptoms, making aspartame the number one source of reported side-effects to the FDA.[84,85]

And what is the number one source of complaints?

Diet soft drinks.[84]

HEALTH ISSUES ASSOCIATED WITH ASPARTAME CONSUMPTION

Regardless of what aspartame proponents claim, study after study—including those known to the manufacturers and sellers of aspartame but hidden from you and me—has shown that if you consistently consume aspartame, you are at risk for a variety of health issues including:[57,59]

- Headaches and migraines—most common symptom
- Chronic fatigue
- Anxiety attacks
- Sleep issues
- Depression
- Vision problems
- Confusion and/or memory loss
- ADD and other behavioral issues
- Obesity…

Obesity??!

Oh, *yes, you can* gain weight by choosing "diet" or "sugar-free." Study after study has shown this to be true.

Artificial sweeteners like aspartame can stimulate your appetite, increase sugar cravings, and promote fat storage.[86-91]
YEEeeehhhaaaawww, where do I sign up??!!

> Aspartame consumption can lead to decreased levels of serotonin in your brain. Serotonin not only influences mood, but also feelings of satiety.[92]

But wait, there's more!

Serious illnesses, which may be triggered or worsened by long-term aspartame consumption include: [59,93,94]

- Brain tumors[95]
- Seizures[81, 96-99]
- Birth defects[31]
- Diabetes: in individuals genetically susceptible to the disease, as well as aggravation of diabetic complications[100-102]
- Various cancers, including leukemia and lymphoma[103-105]
- Neurological disorders (such as autism, multiple sclerosis, Parkinson's, and Alzheimer's)[31,59]

▼ OF EXTREME IMPORTANCE:

Prescription drug interactions may also occur, particularly with anti-depressants!

To report adverse reactions, please go to:

www.fda.gov/Safety/ReportaProblem/ConsumerComplaintCoordinat

ors/default.htm

DOCUMENTARY—*SWEET MISERY: A POISONED WORLD* [106]

Narrator Cori Brackett begins this 2004 documentary with her personal story about consuming Diet Coke® and her subsequent diagnosis with multiple sclerosis. Like many others have reported, she began to recover when she stopped ingesting aspartame.

This movie provides the opinions of several medical experts on the toxic effects of aspartame, while also stating that "aspartame toxicity is the most insidious representation of corporate negligence since tobacco."

Pilots, Seizures, and Aspartame

The Aspartame Consumer Safety Network actually created a hotline for pilots, as many seem to be particularly vulnerable to the effects of aspartame. In fact, abundant toxic reactions have been reported by pilots, including suffering from grand mal seizures in the cockpit.[94]

Whether a result of consuming aspartame at altitude,[107] or merely because pilots may ingest copious amounts of aspartame while flying, warnings about the dangers of aspartame have appeared in a multitude of piloting periodicals (including Australian and British publications), such as:[108-115]

- The Aviation Consumer
- Pacific Flyer
- CAA General Aviation
- Aviation Safety Digest
- General Aviation News
- Plane & Pilot

Additionally, in 1992 the U.S. Air Force magazine, *Flying Safety*, published warnings about aspartame consumption and methanol toxicity, as well as increased vulnerability to seizures, vertigo, and birth defects.[116]

And if all of that was not enough…

Aspartame Is Now on the EPA's List of Neurotoxins

Due to the ever-increasing, astronomical rates of learning disabilities, autism, and neurological disorders, the Environmental Protection Agency (EPA) has been preparing to release a list of chemicals that pose the greatest potential risk to the American public.

And guess what? Aspartame—as well as methanol—has been included on this list, under the category "chemicals with substantial evidence of developmental neurotoxicity."[117]

And Oh No... The Dreaded GMO!

A report by *The Independent (1999)*, revealed that after acquiring the NutraSweet Corporation, biotech giant Monsanto discovered that phenylalanine could be created much more quickly—and probably less expensively—by genetically altering the bacteria required to produce it.[118]

So now, we can add insult-to-injury-ad-infinitum, with aspartame being a union between two of the potentially largest health hazards to ever hit our grocery aisles—artificial sweeteners *and* genetically modified organisms (GMOs).

Aye-yaye-yaye!

SO WHY IS ASPARTAME STILL ON THE SHELVES?

If I have done my job well, the reason is now as clear as the waters of the Caribbean Sea!

But let's do a little recap: Aspartame is still on the shelves because the general public has been duped by political propaganda and skillful marketing fueled by the Diet Industry, which is worth *trillions* of dollars. Corporations want to keep the diet products coming and selling, right alongside the stuff that can make you fat (including aspartame). It's the perfect Corporate-scheming scenario, which, keep in mind, also feeds Big Pharma's coffers. The entire system is the perfect profit-generating machine.

Also, because aspartame has the stamp of GRAS (*generally recognized as safe*) approval, and because the deleterious effects of aspartame are hard to prove—as in a large number of people suddenly dropping dead or falling ill from aspartame-**as-the-linkable-cause**—there is not much motivation for the FDA to remove this potential poison from grocery store shelves. Aspartame simply generates too much cash for all concerned.

The truth is, although some people are violently allergic to aspartame and might know almost immediately, obviously not everyone experiences negative reactions to aspartame. At least not right away. And this can make the association between feeling awful and consuming aspartame very hard to connect. However, as we've learned, the effects of chronic consumption may be cumulative—simply percolating under your skin until one day you feel like crap. What's more, aspartame poisoning can mimic many other health issues and, as a result, is often misdiagnosed as some other disease.[82,93]

So what do you do? If you are concerned, or even just simply pissed off at the way things work, stop buying products made with aspartame. Just remember to keep in mind, if you and your mother and your neighbor and your best friend stop buying aspartame-containing "foods," the Big Boys stop making money. And the Big Boys only make products that fill their pockets with gold. End of story.

▼BE AWARE:

The Corporate Collaborators will most likely create some other inexpensive-to-manufacture-poison to take the rejected product's place. However, you will soon be so savvy in your purchases that you will know to avoid those pitfalls.

In the meantime, keep learning, learning, learning!

🍃 COULD IT BE ASPARTAME?

I have a very close friend who has been drinking copious amounts—think Big Gulps*—of Diet Coke since its inception. Due to my nagging, thank goodness, she has cut back on her daily consumption tremendously (even though she wasn't experiencing any reactions, as far as she knew).

And then just recently, out of nowhere, she developed a fast and irregular heartbeat—a condition known as "atrial fibrillation" (A-fib). It literally feels like the Irish jig is going on in her chest, with episodes sometimes lasting for several disconcerting hours at a time. Although anxiety seems to be one trigger, the A-fib also kicks in randomly, for no apparent reason. And interestingly, she does not fit the bill for the factors that typically cause A-fib. She does not have any kind of heart disease, thyroid issues, or high blood pressure, nor is she a drinker, an endurance athlete, etc.

SOOooooo....might her issue be related to chronic aspartame consumption that is just now presenting symptoms after all these years? Could very well be. Although not the most commonly discussed concern, aspartame has indeed been associated with heart arrhythmias, palpitations, and the like.[77,119,120]

Now if I can just get her to completely abstain from aspartame for just a little while, we may actually solve the mystery and reclaim her heart health.

HOW TO AVOID ASPARTAME

As we learned at the beginning of this chapter, aspartame is an ingredient found in over *6,000* foods and beverages sold worldwide, currently consumed by millions and millions of people *across the globe*.

If you choose to avoid ingesting this insidious ingredient, make sure to search for these various trademarked names—synonymous with aspartame—in the ingredient list of processed foods:

- NutraSweet
- Equal
- Spoonful
- Equal-Measure
- Canderel
- E951
- Naturataste
- Benevia
- AminoSweet (which has been most recently marketed to sound like a healthier alternative)

In Which Products Will I Find Aspartame?

Aspartame is found in more "low-calorie," "diet," "sugar-free," and even "natural" products than you have probably ever imagined, such as:

Cereal, puddings, gelatins, cheesecake, chewing gum, diet soft drinks, chilled juices, powdered soft drinks (think Kool Aid or Crystal Light), dessert mixes, fillings, frozen desserts, yogurt, instant hot cocoa, flavored milk, and tabletop sweeteners. Dairy products of all types have also become an increasingly popular aspartame-carrier, so be on the lookout.

Add to that list: Vitamins, cough drops, children's cough syrup, and various pharmaceuticals. Even the claim "natural flavorings" in an ingredient list can be a sneaky cover for aspartame.

For questions about pharmaceutical ingredients, please check with your pharmacist or read the product inserts for a list of "other" or "inert" ingredients.

▼ BE AWARE:

To reduce the calorie count in unflavored milk, the Dairy Industry has now petitioned the FDA to allow aspartame in milk *without disclosing its presence on the label.*[121] Stay tuned!

THE *BOTTOM* LINE

Our intended judicial system—innocent until proven guilty—seems to apply to food safety as well. Clearly, it should (and is intended to be) the other way around when it comes to things we eat. Like the heavily marketed tobacco tragedy, the American public was repeatedly told it was safe, only to watch people suffer and die from its devastating effects years later. But while smoking is a choice, eating is not. Everyone's gotta eat!

The fact is: To aggressively market *any* product, with knowledge of even *the slightest risk* of severe health implications, is careless, irresponsible, and utterly unethical. Not to mention completely lacking in any kind of compassion whatsoever.

Keep Your Eye on the Champions

As we saw time and again throughout this unbelievable drama, there are many Champions within our Government agencies, as well as the science, medical, and law professions, who do truly care about the good of the whole and doing the right thing. But it's often nearly impossible for these individuals to create positive action when Crooked Corporations are seducing the Official Decision Makers.

The Champions within our system most definitely need our help, support, and appreciation.

THE REALLY GOOD NEWS!

Luckily, no one is forcing aspartame down your throat, so if this information bothered you as much as it did me, you can declare your own personal ban on aspartame. The choice is absolutely, positively yours.

WHAT YOU CAN DO RIGHT NOW

- If your goal is improved health and well-being, please read ingredient lists and avoid aspartame, in all of its many names.

  - ✓ Avoid all "low-calorie," "sugar-free," and "diet" foods. They are full of synthetic, toxic chemicals like aspartame, and they will not help you lose weight.

✓We'll learn more about healthier substitutes in the next book of this series. But for now, I will tell you that my personal favorite is the herb, Stevia (**not** Truvia or PureVia, which are adulterated versions of pure Stevia). It is a safe, natural alternative, but make sure that the brand you choose is made in the U.S., and certified organic, if possible.

As with everything, moderation is key, even with natural sweeteners.

- If you think you or someone you love might be suffering from aspartame toxicity, you can conduct your own experiment.

✓Eliminate **all** aspartame-containing (and all other artificial sweeteners) foods for two weeks.

Then reintroduce aspartame-containing products, one by one, until you reach three servings per day. Give this phase about three days.

If you don't experience any reactions, your body can tolerate aspartame, at least in the short-run.

If you do experience adverse reactions, stop consuming aspartame immediately, and please make sure to report your symptoms to the FDA.

NOTE: Although most people say they can see results in two weeks, it may actually take up to 60 days to see a significant improvement.[122]

- If you feel passionate about getting aspartame off the shelves, or you'd like to learn more, please visit: www.holisticmed.com/aspartame (Aspartame Toxicity Information Center), www.mpwhi.com/main.htm (Mission Possible World Health International), or www.dorway.com (Dorway).

WHAT'S NEXT: BOOK TWO

Aspartame, my friend, is only ONE toxic ingredient of the multitudes circulating throughout our food system that are controlled by Corporations that fully intend to keep them there.

In the next book of this series, we will delve into the topic of processed foods, conventionally produced crops, and GMOs. As always, you will learn how to implement simple solutions to the issues at hand.

We will cover the following subjects, among many others:

- How, backed by Corporate Influence, the government sponsors and encourages the junk food consumption that is making America sick, fat, and tired.

  ✓Why unhealthy food is so damn cheap

  ✓How government funds are allocated and to whom

- What's in your packaged "food"?

  ✓How to read labels

✓ Common label lies, marketing scams, and food fraud

✓ How processed food is *intentionally* created to be addictive

✓ Some of the worst ingredients and foods to avoid and why

- The lowdown on sugar, salt, and fat.

    ✓ The actual villains vs. the true heroes

- The conventional methods of crop production, storage, and processing.

    ✓ The hazards of industrial pesticides/herbicides

    ✓ What's allowed in synthetic fertilizers

    ✓ Irradiation, fumigation, and petrochemicals

And last, but certainly not least, we will tackle (ominous drum roll, please!):

- GMOs

    ✓ What they are

    ✓ The associated health and environmental issues

    ✓ The facts vs. myths

    ✓ How to avoid them

    ✓ A good look at the infamous Monsanto

    ✓ And, of course, how to take action

I look forward to our next adventure!

Until then... be healthy, well, and happy!

"The purpose of government is to enable the people of a nation to live in safety and happiness. Government exists for the interests of the governed, not for the governors."

—THOMAS JEFFERSON

REFERENCES

CHAPTER 1

[1] http://healthreport.saferchemicals.org/ (PDF on website)

[2] America's Children and the Environment: Measures of contaminants, body burdens, and illnesses [Internet]. Washington, DC: Environmental Protection Agency; [updated 2011 March 8]. Available from: www.epa.gov/ace/publications/index.html; www.epa.gov/ace/child_illness/d5-graph.html.

[3] http://www.mountsinai.org/patient-care/service-areas/children/areas-of-care/childrens-environmental-health-center/childrens-disease-and-the-environment.

[4] American Cancer Society, Cancer Facts and Figures 2011. Atlanta: American Cancer Society; 2011. (PDF on website)

[5] http://curechildhoodcancer.ning.com/page/facts-1

[6] State of the Evidence: The connection between breast cancer and the environment [Internet]. San Francisco: Breast Cancer Fund; [2010 October 1]. (PDF on website: "State of the Evidence 2010")

[7] DeSantis C, Ma J, Bryan L, Jemal A. Breast cancer statistics, 2013. *CA Cancer J Clin*. 2014 Jan-Feb;64(1):52-62.

[8] Woodruff T, et al. Trends in environmentally related childhood illnesses. *Pediatrics*, 2004;113(4):1133-1140.

[9] Vital Signs: Asthma prevalence, disease characteristics and self-management education – United States, 2001-2009 [Internet]. Atlanta: U.S. Centers for Disease Control and Prevention Morbidity and Mortality Weekly Report 2011 60(17):547-552; [2011 May 6]. (PDF on Website: "CDC Asthma 2011")

[10] http://home.allergicchild.com/prevalence-of-allergies-in-todays-world/

[11] Boyle C, et al. Trends in the prevalence of developmental disabilities in U.S. children, 1997-2008. *Pediatrics* 2011; 127(6):1034-1042.

[12] Baio, Jon. Centers for Disease Control and Prevention. Prevalence of Autism Spectrum Disorders — Autism and Developmental Disabilities Monitoring Network, 14 Sites, United

States, 2008. Morbidity and Mortality Weekly Report. March 30, 2012. *Surveillance Summaries, March 30, 2012 / 61(SS03); 1-19.* (PDF on website: "Prevalence Autism Spectrum Disorders").

[13] Blumberg, S, Bramlett, M, et al. Changes in Prevalence of Parent-reported Autism Spectrum Disorder in School-aged U.S. Children: 2007 to 2011–2012. National Health Statistics Report, March 2013, Number 65. (PDF on website: Autism Prevalence 2011-2012).

[14] Colborn, T, Soto, A, Von Saal, F. "Developmental Effects of Endocrine-Disrupting Chemicals in Wildlife and Humans," *Environmental Health Perspectives*, Vol. 101, No. 5. October 1993.

[15] Denison R. Ten essential elements in TSCA reform. Environmental Law Review 2009; 39:10020.

[16] Mt Sinai, The Children's Environmental Health Center, Electronic Press Kit. (PDF on website: Mt Sinai chemicals and children's health)

[17] U.S. National Center for Health Statistics, July 31, 2012.

CHAPTER 2

[1] http://www.firstpeople.us/FP-Html-Legends/TwoWolves-Cherokee.html

[2] http://www.forbes.com/largest-private-companies/

[3] Bero LA, Rennie D. Influences on the quality of published drug studies. *Int J Technol Assess Health Care.*1996; 12:209-237.

[4] Rennie D. Thyroid storm. *JAMA.*1997; 277:1238-1243.

[5] Bodenheimer T. Uneasy alliance: clinical investigators and the pharmaceutical industry. *N Engl J Med.* 2000; 342:1539-1544. (PDF on website)

[6] Bekelman JE, Li Y, Gross, CP, et al. MD Scope and Impact of Financial Conflicts of Interest in Biomedical Research: A Systematic Review. *JAMA.* 2003; 289(4):454-465. (PDF on website)

[7] Schulman K, Seils D, Timbie J., et al. A national survey of provisions in clinical-trial agreements between medical schools and industry sponsors. *N Engl J Med.*2002; 347:1335-1341.

[8] Fagin D, Lavelle M, Center for Public Integrity. *Toxic Deception: How the Chemical Industry Manipulates Science, Bends the Law, and Threatens Your Health.* Seacaucus, NJ: Birch Lane Press; 1997:57.

[9] Barnes DE, Bero LA. Why review articles on the health effects of passive smoking reach different conclusions. *JAMA.* 1998; 279:1566–1570.

[10] Lesser LI, Ebbeling CB, Goozner M, Wypij D, Ludwig DS. 2007. Relationship between funding source and conclusion among nutrition-related scientific articles. *Public Library of Science Medicine.* 2007; 4:41-46.

[11] Wazana A. Physicians and the pharmaceutical industry: is a gift ever just a gift? *JAMA.* 2000; 283:373-80.

[12] Kennedy JV. The Sources and Uses of U.S. Science Funding. *The New Atlantis.* 2012; 36:3-22. (PDF on website)

[13] Food & Water Watch, "Public Research, Private Gain: Corporate Influence Over University Agricultural Research." April 2012. (PDF on website). www.foodandwaterwatch.org

[14] Food &Water Watch analysis of Iowa State University grant records obtained through Freedom of Information Act request.

[15] Campbell EG, Weissman JS, Ehringhaus S, et al. Institutional academic-industry relationships. *JAMA.* 2007; 298:1779-86.

[16] Pressman L. *AUTM Licensing Survey, FY 1999: Survey Summary.* Northbrook, Ill: Association of University Technology Managers; 2000.

[17] Nestle, Marion (2001). Food company sponsorship of nutrition research and professional activities: a conflict of interest? *Public Health Nutrition.* 4:1015-1022. (PDF on website: "Food company sponsorship of nutrition research")

[18] Tobacco industry paid scientists to criticize report. *Washington Post.* August 5, 1998:A2.

[19] http://dida.library.ucsf.edu/tid/klc37b10 (PDF on website "Design Write Team")

[20] http://dida.library.ucsf.edu/search?query=Prempro

[21] http://dida.library.ucsf.edu/pdf/amc37b10 (PDF on website "Premarin Family Published Review Papers")

[22] http://dida.library.ucsf.edu/pdf/kjb37b10 (PDF on website "Design Write Business Plan)

[23] http://dida.library.ucsf.edu/tid/eic37b10 (PDF website "Low Dose Publication Plan)

[24] http://dida.library.ucsf.edu/pdf/mtc37b10 (PDF website "Tracking Report")

[25] http://dida.library.ucsf.edu/pdf/lyb37b10 (PDF website "Meeting Agenda")

[26] http://dida.library.ucsf.edu/pdf/fhc37b10 (PDF website "Meeting Minutes")

[27] PDF, courtesy UCSF archives. (on website "dwrite invoice")

[28] http://www.drug-injury.com/drug_injury/prempro/

[29] Rossouw JE, et al. Risks and Benefits of Estrogen Plus Progestin in Healthy

Postmenopausal Women. *JAMA.* 2002; 288(3):321-333.

http://jama.jamanetwork.com/article.aspx?articleid=195120

[30] http://www.druglib.com/ratingsreviews/prempro/

[31] http://acsh.org/category/publications/

[32] http://www.sourcewatch.org/index.php/ACSH

[33] http://tobaccodocuments.org/lor/81210328-0357.html?end_page=30 (PDF on website

"ACSH funding pg 17")

[34] https://s3.amazonaws.com/s3.documentcloud.org/documents/809483/acsh-financial-

summary.pdf (PDF on website "ACSH financial summary" pg 4)

[35] Kroll, Andy, and Jeremy Schulman. "Leaked Documents Reveal the Secret Finances of a

Pro-Industry Science Group." *Mother Jones*, October 28, 2013.

http://www.motherjones.com/politics/2013/10/american-council-science-health-leaked-

documents-fundraising

[36] http://www.cspinet.org/integrity/nonprofits/american_diabetes_association.html

[37] http://www.eatdrinkpolitics.com/wpcontent/uploads/AND_

Corporate_Sponsorship_Report.pdf (PDF on website "AND Corporate Sponsorship Report")

[38] Krimsky S, Rothenberg L. Conflict of interest policies in science and medical journals:

editorial practices and author disclosures. *Sci Eng Ethics.* 2001; 7:205-218.

[39] Hussain A, Smith R. Declaring financial competing interests: survey of five general medical

journals. *BMJ.* 2001; 323:263-264.

[40] Krimsky S, Rothenberg LS, Kyle G, Stott P. Financial interests of authors in scientific

journals: a pilot study of 14 publications. *Sci. Eng. Ethics.* 1996; 2:395-410.

[41] "Stanford's 'Spin' on Organics Allegedly Tainted by Biotechnology Funding." *Cornucopia News,* September 12, 2012. http://www.cornucopia.org/2012/09/stanfords-spin-on-organics-allegedly-tainted-by-biotechnology-funding/

[42] Casadevall A, Fang FC, Steen RG. Misconduct accounts for the majority of retracted scientific publications. *Proc Natl Acad Sci U S A.* 2012 Oct 16; 109(42):17028-33. http://www.ncbi.nlm.nih.gov/pubmed/23027971

[43] http://www.sourcewatch.org/index.php/Portal:Front_groups

[44] Lappé, Anna. *Diet for a Hot Planet:* New York: Bloomsbury, 2010. http://smallplanet.org/

[45] 2011 Tax Return Alliance for Food and Farming (PDF on website)

[46] http://www.sourcewatch.org/index.php?title=Alliance_for_Food_and_Farming#cite_note-CA199-14

[47] http://www.pesticideinfo.org/DCo.jsp?cok=%2700%27

[48] http://www.ewg.org/agmag/2010/09/taxpayers-funding-pro-pesticide-pr-campaign

[49] www.sourcewatch.org/index.php?title=Alliance_for_Food_and_Farming#
Attack_on_the_Environmental_Working_Group
.27s_.22Shoppers_Guide_to_Pesticides_in_Produce.22

[50] http://www.fooddialogues.com/content/affiliates-board-participants-and-industry-partners

[51] Crumb, Michael J. "Farm Groups Form Alliance to Fight Bad Publicity on Animal Welfare, Biotech." *The Huffington Post*, January 31, 2011.
http://www.huffingtonpost.com/2011/02/02/farm-groups-alliance-publicity_n_817510.html

[52] www.foodchaincommunications.com/

[53] http://www.foodchaincommunications.com/joomlaFCC/

[54] http://www.foodchaincommunications.com/index.php?option=com_content&view=article&id=11:bio-kevin-murphy&catid=7&Itemid=21

[55] https://www.facebook.com/CommonGroundNow/info

[56] http://www.sourcewatch.org/index.php/CommonGround#cite_note-2

[57] http://findourcommonground.com/about-us/

[58] http://osbornbarr.com/workbook

[59] http://www.agrimarketing.com/show_story.php?id=23938

[60] http://www.sourcewatch.org/index.php/Osborne_%26_Barr

[61] Martin, A. "Fighting on a Battlefield the Size of a Milk Label." *New York Times* Business section. March 9, 2008.

[62] http://www.whois.com/whois/findourcommonground.com

[63] http://www.consumerfreedom.com/

[64] http://www.consumerfreedom.com/about/

[65] http://www.commoncause.org/site/pp.asp?c=dkLNK1MQIwG&b=6460127

[66] Fischer, Brendan. "PBS Killed Wisconsin Uprising Documentary 'Citizen Koch' To Appease Koch Brothers," *PR Watch*, May 20, 2013. http://www.prwatch.org/news/2013/05/12118/pbs-killed-wisconsin-uprising-documentary-citizen-koch-appease-koch-brothers

[67] Fenn, Peter. "Tea Party Funding Koch Brothers Emerge From Anonymity." *U.S. News*, February 2, 2011. http://www.usnews.com/opinion/blogs/peter-fenn/2011/02/02/tea-party-funding-koch-brothers-emerge-from-anonymity

[68] http://www.forbes.com/forbes-400/

[69] "PBS Killed Wisconsin Uprising Documentary "Citizen Koch" To Appease Koch Brothers." *PR Watch*, May 20, 2013. http://www.prwatch.org/news/2013/05/12118/pbs-killed-wisconsin-uprising-documentary-citizen-koch-appease-koch-brothers

[70] http://www.citizensunited.org/who-we-are.aspx

[71] MacNeal, Caitlin. "Citizens United Constitutional Amendments Introduced In The Senate." *The Huffington Post*, June 19, 2013. http://www.huffingtonpost.com/2013/06/19/citizens-united-constitutional-amendment_n_3465636.html

[72] http://www.opensecrets.org/lobby/index.php

[73] http://www.opensecrets.org/lobby/top.php?indexType=i&showYear=2013

[74] http://www.opensecrets.org/lobby/top.php?indexType=i&showYear=2013

[75] http://www.opensecrets.org/lobby/indus.php?id=A&year=2013

[76] http://www.opensecrets.org/lobby/indusclient.php?id=A09&year=2013

[77] http://www.opensecrets.org/lobby/indusclient.php?id=A07&year=2013

[78] http://www.opensecrets.org/influence/

[79] Fang, Lee. "ANALYSIS: When a Congressman Becomes a Lobbyist, He Gets a 1,452% Raise (on Average)." *Republic Report*, 2012. http://www.republicreport.org/2012/make-it-rain-revolving-door/

[80] http://www.chemheritage.org/Oral-Histories/Documents/TSCA--Fisher--Front-Matter-and-Index.pdf (PDF on website "Linda Fisher career history", pg 4)

[81] http://www.lw.com/industries/LifeSciences

[82] http://www.lightparty.com/Health/BiotechPanel.html

[83] http://www2.dupont.com/Government/en_US/gsa_contracts/our_team/fisher.html

[84] http://www.opensecrets.org/revolving/index.php

[85] http://www.cspinet.org/integrity/about.html

[86] http://www.fda.gov/downloads/AboutFDA/ReportsManualsForms/Reports/BudgetReports/UCM244178.pdf   (on website "FDA Congressional Budget Request)

[87] Federal Register /Vol. 77, No. 148 /Wednesday, August 1, 2012 /Notices: http://www.gpo.gov/fdsys/pkg/FR-2012-08-01/pdf/2012-18711.pdf (PDF on website: "PDUFA FDA user fees")

[88] http://www.opensecrets.org/revolving/search_result.php?agency=Food+%26+Drug+Administration&id=EAHHS09

[89] IMS Health, Press release, 4/20/10.

[90] Mission Possible World Health International, founder Dr. Betty Martini: http://www.mpwhi.com/main.htm

[91] Loudon, Manette. "The FDA Exposed: An Interview With Dr. David Graham, the Vioxx Whistleblower." Natural News, August 30, 2005. http://www.naturalnews.com/011401.html

[92] Budnitz, Daniel S., et al. National Surveillance of Emergency Department Visits for Outpatient Adverse Drug Events. JAMA. 2006; 296(15):1858-1866. http://jama.jamanetwork.com/article.aspx?articleid=203690

[93] US Food and Drug Administration. AERS patient outcomes by year as of December 31, 2008. www.fda.gov/cder/aers/statistics/aers_patient_outcome.htm.

[94] Mayer, Mark H., et al. Reporting Adverse Drug Events. U.S. Pharmacist. 2010; 35:HS-15-HS-19. http://www.uspharmacist.com/content/c/20262/#sthash.Rz6pCdgh.dpuf

[95] Institute for Safe Medicine Practices. "QuarterWatch: Monitoring FDA MedWatch Reports Anticoagulants the Leading Reported Drug Risk in 2011." May 31, 2012. http://www.ismp.org/quarterwatch/pdfs/2011Q4.pdf (PDF on website: "Quarter Watch Drug Report Risks")

[96] http://www.amazon.com/Prescription-Disaster-Gary-Null Production/dp/B000MZXNR0

[97] http://www.citizen.org/hrg1924

[98] http://www.rochester.edu/ORPA/resource/page7box1.html

[99] http://oig.hhs.gov/exclusions/background.asp

[100] Cronin Fisk, Margaret. "U.S. Barred From Prosecuting Off-Label Sales of Drugs." *Bloomberg*, December 4, 2012. http://www.bloomberg.com/news/2012-12-04/u-s-barred-from-prosecuting-off-label-sales-of-drugs.html

[101] Sack, Johnathan. "Law Enforcement In The Health Care Industry: What Do New Cases Against Novartis Tell Us?" *Forbes*, May 9, 2013. http://www.forbes.com/sites/insider/2013/05/09/law-enforcement-in-the-health-care-industry-what-do-new-cases-against-novartis-tell-us/

[102] FDA Science and Mission at Risk: Report of the Subcommittee on Science and Technology." November 2007. http://www.fda.gov/ohrms/dockets/AC/07/briefing/2007-4329b_02_01_FDA%20Report%20on%20Science%20and%20Technology.pdf (PDF on website: "FDA Science and Mission at Risk")

[103] Mercola, Dr. Joseph. "Bayer Buys Schiff for $1.2 Billion." November 14, 2012. http://articles.mercola.com/sites/articles/archive/2012/11/14/bayer-buys-schiff.aspx

[104] Bronstein AC, Spyker DA, Cantilena LR Jr, Green JL, Rumack BH, Dart RC. 2010 Annual Report of the American Association of Poison Control Centers' National Poison Data System (NPDS): 28th Annual Report. *Clinical Toxicology*. 2011 Dec; 49(10):910-41. https://aapcc.s3.amazonaws.com/pdfs/annual_reports/2010_NPDS_Annual_Report_1.pdf

CHAPTER 3

[1] Aspartame, Brain Cancer, & The FDA Approval Process. http://www.youtube.com/watch?v=kn5slnNB8h0

[2] Gold, Mark, 2003. Docket # 02P-0317 *Recall Aspartame as a Neurotoxic Drug: File #7: Aspartame History*, January 2003. (On website: FDA dockets asp as neurotoxic drug #7)

[3] Stoddard, Mary Nash, 1995a. "The Deadly Deception," pg 6. Compiled by the Aspartame Consumer Safety Network for volumes of available published information, ACSN, P.O. Box 780634, Dallas, Texas 75378, (800) 969-6050.

[4] Merrill, Richard, A., 1977. Memorandum from Richard A. Merrill, Chief Counsel, Food and Drug Administration to U.S. Attorney, Samuel K. Skinner, January 10, 1977, Reprinted in Congressional Record 1985b, page S10827-S10835.

[5] Graves, Florence, 1984. "How Safe is Your Diet Soft Drink," Common Cause Magazine, July/August 1984. Reprinted in Congressional Record 1985a, pages S5497-S5506.

[6] Gross, Adrian, 1976b. Memorandum from Mr. Adrian Gross, Scientific Investigations Staff to Mr. Carlton Sharp, Chairman, Searle Investigation Task Force, March 15, 976, Reprinted in U.S. Senate Joint Hearings before the Subcommittee on Health of the Committee on Labor and Public Welfare and the Subcommittee on Administrative Practice and Procedure of the Committee on the Judiciary, "Preclinical and Clinical Testing by the Pharmaceutical Industry, 1976, Part 3," No. Y4.L11/2:P49/2/976/pt.3, CIS# S541-12, page 310-376.

[7] Olney, John W., et al., 1970. "Brain damage in infant mice following oral intake of glutamate, aspartate or cysteine." Nature. 1970; (227):609-610.

[8] Congressional Record 1985a. "Saccharin Study and Labeling Act Amendments of 1985," Volume 131, No. 58, May 7, 1985, page S5489-S5519. (on website)

[9] Farber, Steven A. 1989. "Aspartame and the Regulation of Food Additives: A Study of FDA Decision-Making and a Proposal for Change," Master of Science in Technology and Public Policy Thesis at Massachusetts Institute of Technology, Cambridge, MA 02139.

[10] Federal Register 1974. Volume 39, page 27137.

[11] GAO, 1986. "Six Former HHS Employees' Involvement in Aspartame's Approval," United States General Accounting Office,GAO/HRD-86-109BR, July 1986. (PDF on website "GAO report to Senator Metzenbaum")

[12] Gross, Adrian, 1987. Letter from Dr. Andrian Gross, Former FDA Investigator and Scientist to Senator Howard Metzenbaum regarding pre-approval tests by G.D. Searle, October 30, 1987, Reprinted in US Senate 1987, page 430-439: US Senate 1987. U.S. Senate Committee on Labor and Human Resources, November 3, 1987 regarding "NutraSweet Health and Safety Concerns." Document # Y 4.L11/4:S.HR6.100.

[13] Kennedy, Edward M., 1976. Testimony of U.S. Senator Edward M. Kennedy at the U.S. Senate Joint Hearings before the Subcommittee on Health of the Committee on Labor and Public Welfare and the Subcommittee on Administrative Practice and Procedure of the Committee on the Judiciary, "Preclinical and Clinical Testing by the Pharmaceutical Industry, 1976, Part 3," No. Y4.L11/2:P49/2/976/pt.3, CIS# S541-12, pages 1-2.

[14] Schmidt, Alexander M., 1976c. Statement by Alexander M. Schmidt, Commissioner, U.S. Food and Drug Administration before the U.S. Senate Joint Hearings before the Subcommittee on Health of the Committee on Labor and Public Welfare and the Subcommittee on Administrative Practice and Procedure of the Committee on the Judiciary, "Preclinical and Clinical Testing by the Pharmaceutical Industry, 1976, Part 3," No. Y4.L11/2:P49/2/976/pt.3, CIS# S541-12, page 3-56.

[15] Buzzard, James A., 1976a. Testimony of James A. Buzzard, G.D. Searle, before the U.S. Senate Joint Hearings before the Subcommittee on Health of the Committee on Labor and Public Welfare and the Subcommittee on Administrative Practice and Procedure of the Committee on the Judiciary, "Preclinical and Clinical Testing by the Pharmaceutical Industry, 1976, Part 2," No. Y4.L11/2:P49/2/976/pt2, CIS# S541-82, page 168

[16] Gordon, Gregory, 1987. "NutraSweet: Questions Swirl," UPI Investigative Report, 3-part series. 10/12/87. Reprinted in U.S. Senate Committee on Labor and Human Resources, November 3, 1987 regarding "NutraSweet Health and Safety Concerns." Document # Y 4.L 11/4:S.HR6.100, pages 483-510. (On website)

[17] *The Journal of Toxicology and Environmental Health: Volume 2, Issue 2, 1976.*

- http://www.tandfonline.com/doi/abs/10.1080/15287397609529442#.UzWIpc5Wz0c
- http://www.tandfonline.com/doi/abs/10.1080/15287397609529443#.UzWI985Wz0c
- http://www.tandfonline.com/doi/abs/10.1080/15287397609529444#.UzWJLs5Wz0c
- http://www.tandfonline.com/doi/abs/10.1080/15287397609529445#.UzWJYM5Wz0c
- http://www.tandfonline.com/doi/abs/10.1080/15287397609529446#.UzWJoM5Wz0c
- http://www.tandfonline.com/doi/abs/10.1080/15287397609529448#.UzWJ4s5Wz0c

[18] Gross, Adrian, 1985. Statement from Dr. Adrian Gross, Former FDA Investigator and Scientist, "Aspartame Safety Act," Congressional Record, Volume 131, No. 106, August 1, 1985, page S10835-S10840.

[19] Mullarkey, Barbara, 1994b. Account of John Cook as published in Informed Consent Magazine. "How Safe Is Your Artificial Sweetener" by Barbara Mullarkey, September/October 1994. Available from Informed Consent Magazine, P.O. Box 935, Williston, ND 58802-0935, 701/859- 3002. Available from NutriVoice, P.O. Box 946, Oak Park, Illinois 60303, (708) 848-0116.

[20] http://en.wikipedia.org/wiki/Donald_Rumsfeld

[21] Verrett, Jacqueline, 1987. Statement of Dr. Jacqueline Verrett, Former Toxicologist, U.S. Food and Drug Administration before U.S. Senate Committee on Labor and Human Resources, November 3, 1987 regarding "NutraSweet Health and Safety Concerns." Document # Y 4.L11/4:S.HR6.100, page 383-390.

[22] Bressler Report (FDA Investigation). Complete report on website.

[23] Discussion of Bressler Report available on Page 497 of US Senate 1987. U.S. Senate Committee on Labor and Human Resources, November 3, 1987 regarding "NutraSweet Health and Safety Concerns." Document # Y 4.L 11/4:S.HR6.100.

[24] Gross, Adrian, 1987b. Letter from Dr. Andrian Gross, Former FDA Investigator and Scientist to Senator Howard Metzenbaum regarding pre-approval tests by G.D. Searle, November 3, 1987, page 2-5.Reprinted in US Senate 1987, page 443-453.

[25] Olney, John W. 1987. Letter from Dr. John W. Olney, Neuropathologis, Washington University School of Medicine, to Senator Howard M. Metzenbaum, December 8, 1987, page 6-7. Presented in the record before the U.S. Senate Committee on Labor and Human Resources, November 3, 1987 regarding "NutraSweet Health and Safety Concerns." Document # Y 4.L 11/4:S.HR6.100, page 468-476.

[26] Federal Register 1979. "Ruling on Objections and Notice of Hearing Before a Public Board of Inquiry; Aspartame," Federal Register, Volume 44, page 31,717.

[27] Federal Register 1981. "Aspartame: Commissioner's Final Decision," Federal Register, Volume 46, page 38284-38308.

[28] Letter to Betty Martini from Linda Hart, Goyan's widow. (PDF on website)

[29] Sveda, Michael. "Cyclamate." Diabetes Daily. http://www.diabetesdaily.com/wiki/Cyclamate

[30] http://www.fda.gov/Food/FoodIngredientsPackaging/FoodAdditives/ucm082418.htm (first referenced here, when status was "held in abeyance") **Current:**

http://www.fda.gov/Food/IngredientsPackagingLabeling/FoodAdditivesIngredients/ucm091048.htm#ftnC

[31] Monte, Woodrow. "While Science Sleeps: A Sweetener Kills." San Francisco: Amazon Create Space Publishing, 2011. http://www.whilesciencesleeps.com/

[32] US Senate 1987. U.S. Senate Committee on Labor and Human Resources, November 3, 1987 regarding "NutraSweet Health and Safety Concerns." Document # Y 4.L 11/4:S.HR6.100. Pages 483-510.

[33] Congressional Record 1982. "Orphan Drug Act," Congressional Record, December 14, 1982, page 30445.

[34] Federal Register 1983. "Food Additives Permitted for Direct Addition to Food: Aspartame," 48(July 8): 31376-31382.

[35] Metzenbaum, Senator Howard, 1985. Testimony of U.S. Senator Howard Metzenbaum of Ohio at "Aspartame Safety Act," Congressional Record, Volume 131, No. 106, August 1,1985, page S10821.

[36] Federal Register 1984. "Food Additives Permitted for Direct Addition to Food for Human Consumption; Aspartame," Volume 49, No. 36, February 22, 1984, page 6672-6682.

[37] Shiver, Jube Jr. "Monsanto to Acquire G. D. Searle & Co. in $2.7-Billion Cash Deal." *Los Angeles Times*, July 19, 1985.
http://articles.latimes.com/1985-07-19/business/fi-6792_1_searle-family

[38] "Winter comes for a Beltway lion; Rumsfeld rose and fell with his conviction intact." *Chicago Tribune*: p. 17. November 12, 2006.

[39] www.sourcewatch.org/index.php?title=International_Life_Sciences_Institute

[40] http://www.wnho.net/congressionalrecord.htm

[41] USDA, 1988. "1988 United States Department of Agriculture Situation and Outlook Report; Sugar and Sweeteners." Washington, DC: U.S. Government Printing Office, pp. 51.

[42] GAO 1987. "Food Additive Approval Process Followed for Aspartame," United States General Accounting Office, GAO/HRD-87-46, June 1987. (PDF on website "FDA and GAO Review")

[43] GAO 2009. "The Role of The U.S. Government Accountability Office," United States Accountability Office, GAO-10-111CG, October 2009. (PDF on website "GAO Mission")

[44] Office of Pollution Prevention and Toxics, U.S. ENVIRONMENTAL PROTECTION AGENCY, Chemical Summary for Methanol. August 1994. http://www.epa.gov/chemfact/f_methan.txt

[45] International Agency for Research on Cancer (IARC). Agents Classified by the *IARC Monographs*, Volumes 1 – 100. 2011. http://monographs.iarc.fr/ENG/Classification/ClassificationsGroupOrder.pdf

[46] www.cancer.org/cancer/cancercauses/othercarcinogens/ generalinformationaboutcarcinogens/known-and-probable-human-carcinogens

[47] ACGIH. 1991. American Conference of Governmental Industrial Hygienists, Inc. Documentation of the Threshold Limit Values and Biological Exposure Indices, 6th ed., pp. 903-905.

[48] Roe, O. Species Differences in Methanol Poisoning. I. Minimal Lethal Doses. Symptoms. And Toxic Sequelae of Methanol Poisoning in Humans and Experimental Animals. *CRC Critical Reviews in Toxicology.* 1982;18:376-90

[49] Trocho C, Pardo R, Fafecas I, Virgili J, Remesar X, Fernandez-Lopez JA, et al. Formaldehyde derived from dietary aspartame binds to tissue components in vivo. *Life Sci.* 1988; 63(5):337-49.

[50] http://www.whilesciencesleeps.com/methanol/

[51] Cleland, J.G. and Kingsbury, G.L., Multimedia Environmental Goals For Environmental Assessment. U.S. Environmental Protection Agency: EPA-600/7-77-136b, E-28, November 1977.

[52] "FDA Finding on Aspartame," *New York Times*, January 14, 1984, p. 28.

[53] Monte, Dr. Woodrow C. Aspartame: methanol, and the public health. *Journal of Applied Nutrition* 1984; 36(1): 42-54. http://www.whilesciencesleeps.com/pdf/1.pdf

[54] Ekins B, Duffy D, Gregory M, and Rollins, D. Standardized Treatment of Severe Methanol Poisoning With Ethanol and Hemodialysis. *West J Med.* Mar 1985; 142(3): 337–340. www.ncbi.nlm.nih.gov/pmc/articles/PMC1306022/

[55] Oppermann, J.A., Muldoon, E. and Ranney, R.E. Metabolism of Aspartame in Monkey. *J. Nutr.* 1973; 103:1454-1459.

[56] Zatmann, L.J. The Effect of Ethanol on the Metabolism of Methanol in Man. *Biochem. J.* 1946; 40:67-68.

[57] Gold, Mark, 2002. Docket # 02P-0317 *Recall Aspartame as a Neurotoxic Drug: File #1*: Aspartame History, January 2002.

http://www.fda.gov/ohrms/DOCKETS/dailys/03/Jan03/012203/02P-0317_emc-000196.txt

[58] Gruner, O and Bilzer, N. Methanol content of fruit-juices. Its significance in congener analysis. *Blutalkohol.* 1983; 20:241.

[59] Roberts, H.J. *Aspartame Disease: An Ignored Epidemic*. West Palm Beach, Sunshine Sentinel Press. May 2001.

[60] Pattanaargson S, Sanchavanakit C. Aspartame degradation study using electrospray ionization mass spectrometry. *Rapid Commun. Mass Spectrom.* 2000; 14(11), 987-93.

[61] Olney JW, Farber NB, Spitznagel E, Robins LN. Increasing brain tumor rates: is there a link to aspartame? *J. Neuropathol. Exp. Neurol.* Nov 1996; 55(11): 1115–23.

[62] Shephard SE, Wakabayashi K, Nagao M. Mutagenic activity of peptides and the artificial sweetener aspartame after nitrosation. *Food and Chemical Toxicology: an international journal published for the British Industrial Biological Research Association.* May 1993; 31(5): 323–9.

[63] JECFA, Toxicological evaluation of certain food additives: aspartame, WHO food additive series No 15, Report series No 653, 1980.

[64] Walton, Ralph G. M.D. Survey of Aspartame Studies: Correlation of Outcome and Funding Sources. (PDF on website: "Dr. Walton Survey of Aspartame Studies")

[65] Food & Water Watch, "Public Research, Private Gain: Corporate Influence Over University Agricultural Research." April 2012. (PDF on website: "Buying Universities"). www.foodandwaterwatch.org

[66] http://www.cspinet.org/integrity/corp_funding.html

[67] http://www.coca-colacompany.com/coca-cola-unbottled/hitting-the-sweet-spot

[68] http://www.cancer.org/cancer/cancercauses/othercarcinogens/athome/aspartame

[69] http://www.cancer.org/aboutus/honoringpeoplewhoaremakingadifference/corporations/corporations-corporate-donations

[70] http://www.sourcewatch.org/index.php/American_Cancer_Society

[71] www.caloriecontrol.org

[72] http://www.caloriecontrol.org/about-the-council

[73] http://www.kellenpr.com/

[74] http://www.kellencompany.com/companies/what-we-do/public-relations

[75] http://www.kellencommunications.com/about.asp

[76] http://www.nutrasweet.com/articles/category.asp?lev1=Links&lev2=Industry+Organizations

[77] Gold, Mark. Docket # 02P-0317 *Recall Aspartame as a Neurotoxic Drug: File #4: Reported Aspartame Toxicity Reactions*. January 2003. (On website: "ASP toxicity reactions")

[78] Kessler, David A. Introducing MEDWatch: A New Approach to Reporting Medication and Device Adverse Effects and Product Problems. *Journal of the American Medical Association.* 1993; 269:2765-68.

[79] Food 1995. "Aspartame Adverse Reaction Reports Down in 1994 From 1985 Peak: FDA." *Food Chemical News.* June 12, 1995, page 27.

[80] Turner, James, Leonard, Rodney. Letter from Rodney E. Leonard and James S. Turner of Community Nutrition Institute to Dr. Fank E. Young, FDA Commissioner, September 13, 1984. Reprinted in "Aspartame Safety Act," Congressional Record, Volume 131, No. 106.

[81] Turner, James. Testimony of James Turner, Esq., Community Nutrition Institute before the U.S. Senate Committee on Labor and Human Resources, November 3, 1987 regarding "NutraSweet Health and Safety Concerns." Document # Y 4.L 11/4:S.HR6.100, page 316.

[82] Pauli, George. FDA Center for Food Safety and Applied Nutrition (CFSAN). Radio broadcast: "Aspartame," The Derek McGinty Show, WAMU Radio (88.5 FM), Brandywine Building, The American University, Washington, DC 20016- 8082, (202) 885-1200, August 29, 1995.

[83] Butchko, Harriett H., Kotsonis, Frank N. "Postmarketing Surveillance in the Food Industry: The Aspartame Case Study," in *Nutritional Toxicology*, edited by Frank N. Kotsonis, Maureen Macky and Jerry Hjelle, Raven Press, Ltd., New York, c1994.

[84] DHHS. "Summary of Adverse Reactions Attributed to Aspartame," Department of Health and Human Services. Documents dated 1995, 1996, and 1997. Obtained by Dr. Betty Martini through Freedom of Information Act. (PDF on website: "DHHS report 92 Aspartame Symptoms").

[85] Roberts, H.J., 1988. Reactions Attributed to Aspartame- Containing Products: 551 Cases. *Journal of Applied Nutrition*. 1988; 40:85-94.

[86] Gropper, George. *Biochemistry of Human Nutrition*. Wadsworth, Inc. 2000.

[87] Davidson TL, Swithers SE. A Pavlovian approach to the problem of obesity. *Int J Obes Relat Metab Disord*. July 2004; 28(7):933-5.

[88] Yang, Q. Gain weight by 'going diet?' Artificial sweeteners and the neurobiology of sugar cravings. *Yale J Biol Med*. Jun 2010; 83(2): 101–108. http://www.ncbi.nlm.nih.gov/pmc/articles/PMC2892765/

[89] Feijó, Fernanda de Matos, et al. Saccharin and aspartame, compared with sucrose, induce greater weight gain in adult Wistar rats, at similar total caloric intake levels. *Appetite*. January 1, 2012; 60: 203-207. http://www.sciencedirect.com/science/article/pii/S0195666312004138

[90] Davidson, TL, Swithers, SE. A role for sweet taste: calorie predictive relations in energy regulation by rats. *Behavioral Neuroscience*. 2008 Feb; 122(1):161-73. http://www.ncbi.nlm.nih.gov/pubmed/18298259

[91] UT Health Center San Antonio Press Release, "New analysis suggests 'diet soda paradox' – less sugar, more weight." June 14, 2005 · Volume: XXXVIII · Issue: 24. http://uthscsa.edu/hscnews/singleformat2.asp?newID=1539

[92] H. L. Wang, V. H. Harwalkar and H. A. Waisman. Effect of dietary phenylalanine and tryptophan on brain serotonin. *Archives of Biochemistry and Biophysics* April 1962; 97(1): 181-184.

[93] Mission Possible 1994. Compiled by researchers, physicians, and artificial sweetener experts for Mission Possible, a group dedicated to warning consumers about aspartame. Available from Mission Possible, 9270 River Club Pkwy, Duluth, Georgia 30155, 770-242-2599, betty@pd.org.

[94] Stoddard, Mary Nash, 1995. Conversations between Mary Nash Stoddard of the Aspartame Consumer Safety Network and Mark D. Gold.

[95] Olney JW, Farber NB, Spitznagel E, Robins LN. Increasing brain tumor rates: is there a link to aspartame? *J Neuropathol Exp Neurol*. 1996 Nov; 55(11):1115-23.

[96] *Food Chemical News*, July 28, 1986, page 44.

[97] Wurtman, Richard J., 1985. "Aspartame: Possible Effect on Seizure Susceptibility," *The Lancet*, Volume 2, page 1060.

[98] Walton, Ralph G. Seizure and Mania After High Intake of Aspartame. *Psychosomatics*, 1986; 27: 218-220.

[99] Walton, Ralph G., 1988. "The Possible Role of Aspartame in Seizure Induction," Presented at "Dietary Phenylalanine and Brain Function." Proceedings of the First International Meeting on Dietary Phenylalanine and Brain Function, Washington, D.C., May 8-10, 1987. Center for Brain Sciences and Metabolism Charitable Trust, P.O. Box 64, Kendall Square, Cambridge, MA 02142. Reprinted in "Dietary Phenyalalnine and Brain Function," c1988, Birkhauser, Boston, MA USA, page 159-162.

[100] Roberts, HJ. The Trouble with Sweeteners - Artificial Sweeteners, the Pancreas and Diabetes. *Nutrition Health Review*. Spring 2003.

[101] Blaylock. R.L. *Excitotoxins: The Taste That Kills*. Santa Fe, NM: Health Press 1994.

[102] Statement of H.J. Roberts, M.D. Concerning the Use of Products Containing Aspartame (Nutrasweet) by Persons with Diabetes and Hypoglycemia.
http://www.dorway.com/diabetes.txt

[103] Soffritti M, Belpoggi F, Esposti D, Lambertini L, Tibaldi E, Rigano A. First Experimental Demonstration of the Multipotential Carcinogenic Effects of Aspartame Administered in the Feed to Sprague-Dawley Rats. *Environmental Health Perspectives*. March 2006; 114(3):379-85.

[104] Soffritti M, Belpoggi F, Tibaldi E, Esposti DD, Lauriola M. Life-span exposure to low doses of aspartame beginning during prenatal life increases cancer effects in rats. *Environmental Health Perspectives*. September 2007; 115(9):1293-7.

[105] Schernhammer ES, Bertrand KA, Birmann BM, Sampson L, Willett WC, Feskanich D. Consumption of artificial sweetener- and sugar-containing soda and risk of lymphoma and leukemia in men and women. *Am J Clin Nutr*. 2012 Dec; 96(6):1419-28. Epub 2012 Oct 24.

[106] *Sweet Misery: A Poisoned World*. 2005. http://www.amazon.com/Sweet-Misery-A-Poisoned-World/dp/B000BQ5IWS

[107] Moskal, Phil, 1990. Letter from Dr. Phil Moskal to George Leighton, June 19, 1990, Reprinted in "The Deadly Deception" Compiled by the Aspartame Consumer Safety Network

for volumes of available published information, ACSN, P.O. Box 780634, Dallas, Texas 75378, (800) 969-6050.

[108] Aviation Consumer 1988. "SafeGuard." June 15, 1988.

[109] Aviation Medical Bulletin 1988. "Pilots and Aspartame." October 1988.

[110] Pacific Flyer 1995. "ICAS Issues Warning To Its Members About Diet Drinks." March 1995.

[111] Pacific Flyer 1988. "This Could Save Your Life." *Pacific Flyer Aviation News*, November 1988, 3355 Mission Ave., Oceanside, CA 92054.

[112] CAA General Aviation (1989). Safety Information Leaflet, April 1989, Great Britain.

[113] Aviation Safety Digest 1989. "Aspartame -- not for the dieting pilot?" *Aviation Safety Digest*, ASD 142, Spring 1989. (Australia - 062/5841111).

[114] Hicks, Megan. "NutraSweet...too good to be true?" *General Aviation News*. July 31, 1989.

[115] Plane & Pilot. "Getting High." *Plane & Pilot*. January 1990, page 36-37.

[116] US Air Force 1992. "Aspartame Alert." *Flying Safety*. . May 1992. 48(5): 20-21

[117] http://www.epa.gov/ncct/toxcast/files/summit/48P%20Mundy%20TDAS.pdf (on website: "EPA List of Neurotoxic Chemicals")

[118] Wolff, Marie. "World's top sweetener is made with GM bacteria." *The Independent*. June 20, 1999.

http://www.independent.co.uk/news/worlds-top-sweetener-is-made-with-gm-bacteria-1101176.html

[119] Roberts, H.J. "Aspartame Induced Arrhythmias and Sudden Death." 2004.

http://www.wnho.net/aspartame_and_arrhythmias.htm

[120] Burkhart, Craig G. "Lone atrial fibrillation precipitated by MSG and Aspartame." *OpEdNews*. December 10, 2009.

http://www.opednews.com/articles/--Lone-atrial-fibrillati-by-Craig-G-Burkhart-091207-399.html

[121] Federal Register, Proposed rule February 20, 2013. Flavored Milk; Petition to Amend the Standard of Identity for Milk and 17 Additional Dairy Products.

https://www.federalregister.gov/articles/2013/02/20/2013-03835/flavored-milk-petition-to-amend-the-standard-of-identity-for-milk-and-17-additional-dairy-products

[122] http://www.holisticmed.com/aspartame/

Made in the USA
Lexington, KY
23 December 2014